—A SPIRITUAL—
PREGNANCY

—A SPIRITUAL—
PREGNANCY

22 Ways to Connect With Your Unborn Child.

Catherine Sweet

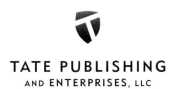

TATE PUBLISHING
AND ENTERPRISES, LLC

Published by Tate Publishing & Enterprises, LLC
127 E. Trade Center Terrace | Mustang, Oklahoma 73064 USA
1.888.361.9473 | www.tatepublishing.com

Tate Publishing is committed to excellence in the publishing industry. The company reflects the philosophy established by the founders, based on Psalm 68:11,
"The Lord gave the word and great was the company of those who published it."

Book design copyright © 2015 by Tate Publishing, LLC. All rights reserved.
Cover design by Ivan Charlem Igot
Interior design by Gram Telen

Published in the United States of America

ISBN: 978-1-63367-488-2
1. Health & Fitness / Pregnancy & Childbirth
2. Body, Mind & Spirit / Spiritualism
15.01.27

To God, Christ, and the Holy Spirit, for a journey of the soul that we are blessed as women to experience.

To Gary, who completes my life with love, joy, kindness, and caring. Thank you for creating each day as a special gift.

To my wonderful family and friends who have been supporting me on this journey of life.

To the love of Christ in each of us.

Acknowledgments

Thank you, Holy Spirit, for your gift of guidance. Thank you to the ageless spirit of humanity that seeks the truth of our identity. Thank you to my father and mother who devoted their lives to their children. Thank you, Tate Publishing, for working with me to create a spiritual book. Thank you, Carolyn Stanley, for your technical help in creating a workable manuscript. Thank you for the women who bring children into this world to know God.

Contents

Introduction

When I was pregnant, I had a special spiritual bonding with our unborn child. At that time, I felt a need for the sacredness of pregnancy to be available to everyone. Through prayer and my belief in Christ, I feel I was guided to write this simple book to honor our spiritual journey. The world seems to be pulling away from our ancient past and our spiritual beginnings. At this special time in your life, let yourself explore the gentler subtle energies of nature. These energies of nature bring each of us closer to God our Creator. I am grateful for sharing these lessons that connect you to spirit, and I hope they will bring your pregnancy closer to God.

Pregnancy is a new beginning of life. This journey is beyond the physical world. This journey is sacred.

Pregnancy is a spiritual, physical, emotional, and mental passage. As parents, you are both involved in a spiritual journey together, and you will be experiencing the subtle energy of your unborn child's consciousness.

To begin spiritual communication, you must quiet yourself and listen to sense the subtle energies that surround you. These lessons allow you to explore the subtle energies of life and teach you how to sense the spiritual essence of these different forms of life.

By creating a sacred space in your home, you can focus a busy mind and surround yourself with an environment of peace and safety for your unborn child. Through peace and prayer, you can connect with this special child, who has been sent by God.

Communing with nature and its subtle energies gives you and your family a hint of the energies of your unborn child. Sensing the subtle energy of plants and rocks is a method of sensing the energy of the unmanifest spirit.

In these gentle lessons, you will explore the spiritual intimacy of motherhood and the ancient folklore of our distant ancestors. Lessons include visualizations, relaxing baths, prayers, auric energies, ancient sacred maps, and easy exercises to unite you with the spirit of your unborn child. Let your pregnancy be a spiritual experience and not just a physical journey.

Let your family be involved with this sacred experience. Learn about sacred sounds and music that can feed the soul. Walk the mystical paths of labyrinths that historically were a form of divining and meditation that brings the body and mind into peace. Walking a sacred path brings you and your child into another experience of spiritual closeness.

There is a divine origin of music. Sacred languages of Hebrew and Sanskrit have a special property. When we speak them, they create form! There is a corresponding numerology to musical notes, and with a simple chart, you can create the melody of the name you are choosing for your unborn child.

The Chinese, centuries ago, have corresponded musical notes and sounds to health. There are six yin organs and six yang organs. There are lessons that bring the family into a musical meditation that tones a note to send harmonious energy to the organs that are being formed in the womb.

There are feelings and emotions that, centuries ago, were labeled by the Chinese to relate to organs. These tones and sounds will bring you and your unborn child into the sacred space of creation through music.

Singing gentle lullabies to your child brings them emotional peace and creates a bond that the child associates with safety and love. The philosophy of lullabies and classical music and how it is the same beat as our heart creates a physical harmony in our tissue. We sing because our spirit interacts with our emotional bodies. The blues draw you to sadness; gospel enlivens your soul and expresses hope and faith. The lullabies bring us to a rhythmic calm. Music is greater than the feeling it brings; music interacts with our cells.

The breath of life restores your tissue, your subtle energies, and your link to God with each breath. There are exercises to harmonize, detoxify, and enliven you and your unborn child with the breath of life.

Guiding Angels are surrounding you and your child at this time. In the ancient text of Kabbalah, there is a philosophy that maps the Angelic Hosts and their purpose. In meditation, you can understand the ancient journey that describes the interaction of the Angelic Hosts and your unborn child as spirit creates life.

In myth and astrology, our passage at birth, through a constellation, interacts with our process in this world. These constellations were also described in the Old Testament. This idea is an ancient journey through the heavens to earth at birth.

As we honor our closeness to God, Christ, and the Holy Spirit, the holy names of God bring us to a level of spiritual communication that is between our soul and God consciousness. To meditate and sound the names of God brings that consciousness into our planet. The energy of billions of people for thousands of years praying each day, all over the world, creates a mass of energy of God consciousness that brings you to feel the subtle energy of your human spirit. Bring the consciousness of God to your unborn child by praying intently with the sacred name of God.

In the Bible, there are gifts of the Holy Spirit that are given to each soul at conception. Experience visualization as a confirmation of these gifts for your unborn child.

Your pathway is a sacred one that is involved in spiritual evolution. The oneness of spirit links everyone together in a consciousness of God. Feel through these lessons, exercises, prayers, and meditations how we are truly one in the body of Christ. Be joyful for your sacred gift of life.

What Is Spirit?

Lesson 1
Spirit Creates Consciousness

Life is the breath of spirit that moves like a wave through each cell of your body. This wave of energy flows in and out, creating physical tissue, thoughts, and actions.

The breath of spirit begins when consciousness of two become one. In the sacred space where the egg and sperm unite, at that moment, the energy shifts and creation begins.

The replicating DNA, given lovingly by each parent, manifests a new essence of spirit. This new essence of spirit also contains the memories of past generations. The history of consciousness is in our genes. The past lives of our ancestors have blessed us with evolving consciousness and understanding that expresses itself as better health care, more spiritual consciousness, and a greater understanding of science and our world. This results in knowledge of how we interact to create a whole ecosystem and how we perceive ourselves. The consciousness carried in the nucleus of the cell moves through time, creating a consciousness of humanity that makes us all one.

In this oneness of sacred energy, the Creator of all things guides our every breath. This sacred energy of God, as a wave of light, brings consciousness into physical form. This energy of the Creator congeals into life. It touches upon the light electromagnetic system of acupuncture and passes into denser neurological tissue then creates glandular tissue, muscle, organ, and, finally—the densest—bone. The passage of the unmanifest spirit into life is the same passage lightning takes when it strikes an individual. When our thoughts create disharmonious energies of disease, this energy follows this same route through our tissues, deep into our bones.

During these nine months, the energy of life that permeates matter and creates your child is not only physical energy. It is the embodiment of spirit in form. It is the energy of thought (mental body), the energy of feeling (emotional body), and the energy of oneness (spiritual body–God consciousness).

As your child emerges at birth, all these bodies are just as they are inside of you as an adult.

Your ability to think did not enter on the first day of school, nor did your ability to feel the first time you cut yourself.

You are a spiritual, an emotional, and a mental being in a physical body. Your bodies are interconnected and create a whole being.

As the parent, you are the conduit of sacred space. A space that allows that child's innermost will to flourish. A sacred space that allows thought, action, and feeling to enter into that child's essence. God has created this perfect being to come to earth with a special purpose. It may be to become a doctor or to save someone from a fire (fireman). We are all one in consciousness, and we interlink to create a whole. We are part of the body of Christ. Each child is important, and their will and destiny is a vital part of the manifestation of spirit. As a parent, you try to create this space in your home. As a spiritually conscious parent, you try to create this space in your womb.

Every religious philosophy describes a spark of light that is the essence of God. This Holy Spirit penetrates every cell in our bodies, linking us to God consciousness. These lessons are about that spark of light, the essence of God that flows through all living beings. The Holy Spirit is the connection we have to the divine. These lessons teach you how to experience and understand that subtle energy of life that connects your Holy Spirit to that divine spark of life that penetrates your womb.

Lesson 2
Creating a Sacred Space

Motherhood is a sacred passage. Creating a special time and space to communicate with your child is important. Being comfortable, acknowledging your special worth, and having a closeness to the Spirit during these nine months will help you begin this journey. This lesson will help you to get started.

The approach to this book is one of peace, contemplation, and meditation. Set aside a quiet time with yourself and your unborn child; involve your husband and other children when at all possible. Use these moments to daily communicate with your child and his or her spirit. Always stroke your lower abdomen gently while you talk to your baby. Keep in mind that this baby is spiritually a conscious being, conscious of your joys and your sorrows.

Try to place yourself and your child in a quiet warm room. It is important to put your mind at peace, to open your other senses to the subtle energies of life. Prepare your surroundings to respect the sacredness of your journey. The child that you carry is floating in a warm soft fluid, being bathed always in your energy and the love that flows from your heart.

To create a sacred space in your home, think of creating a beautiful energetic environment. Begin to sense the feeling of life rather than evaluating life through sight. If we close our eyes, we begin to sense that feeling of life.

Place a Candle in Your Space

Light a candle in your peaceful place. As the light fills the room, you can feel the connections of ancient archetypes that express us as beings of light. The science of the twentieth century brings this energy of life into truth. The famous equation $E=mc^2$ relates energy (E) to matter (m) to (c) the speed of light squared. All that we see as matter and form and all that we feel as energy are related to the waves of light that pour into your room, touching your skin.

Place a Flower in Your Space

A flower or plant brings life into a room. If you have a flowering plant, notice its shape and colors. Try to feel the energy that surrounds the plant. Their continuous release of oxygen supplies your environment with necessary molecular nutrients. With every breath we take, we connect to the spirit of the life force within us. Each breath, twelve to sixteen times a minute, floods a wave of energy that rises in our spine and travels along our nerves, bathing our brain in life. This rhythmic tide cannot flourish in stale air. The sense of subtle energy is truly the sense of our interrelationship with the plant kingdom.

Place a Special Rock in Your Space

Rocks are alive with energy! Rocks are made of elements that are also found in our bones and tissue. They create the ground we walk on. The crust of the earth is mostly silicates (sand quartz). When a metal infuses into the lattice structure of quartz, we wear it on our finger as an amethyst, topaz, opal, zircon, or garnet (quartz silicates). Different waves of light are absorbed into the tissue and structure of the rocks. What we perceive is reflected back to interact with our molecular levels of tissue and consciousness. Each colored stone has an inherent personality of waveforms that subtly interact with our energy.

There are magnetic, electrical, and radioactive rocks. Magnetic rocks attract iron (magnetite), and piezoelectric rocks (quartz), upon being squeezed, produce currents that run our watches. Microchips of silicone have helped to develop and evolve our computer systems.

Radioactive rocks are continually spewing out nuclear particles; they are molecularly alive and producing waste! Radioactivity has allowed us to develop x-rays, which have helped millions.

Certain minerals, when placed under ultraviolet light, will glow an incredible iridescent color, like an aura. They are said to fluoresce.

Just as we trace our ancestors before us, rocks also have kept historical records. These fossils record the life history of the earth. The formation of plants and animals and the passage of ancient footprints are recorded in fossil rocks. Dinosaurs are a popular name for a large group of fossils.

Lava rocks are thrown out of the earth during earthquakes. They are rough and filled with air pockets.

Meteorites are extraterrestrial in origin and generally fragmented and angular due to collisions. They are the solid matter of our solar system, and they tell the story of the composition and early history of the interior of our planet. Meteorites come from that same energetic universe that the spirit of your unborn child has come from: the energy of the heavens.

Sacred rocks are found in prehistoric structures like Stonehenge, England. In England, there is a special coronation rock under the king's throne; without, it coronations would not be considered valid.

There are so many different energies and personalities in the mineral kingdom that to choose a rock for your sacred space is difficult. To honor the unique energies of the mineral kingdom honors your relationship to nature and our universe. God, the Creator of all things, created the mineral kingdom.

Bring a rock into your sacred space. Whether it be a meteorite from the heavens—as your child's heaven sent—or a rock from your yard, each has the sacred energy of the Creator. It will enhance the energy of your space.

Bring in a Favorite Photo

In your sacred space, you may bring in photos of loved ones or religious paintings. This will bring you loving thoughts that will fill the room with happiness. Consciousness and intention are the most important part of the understanding of subtle energy. Be vigilant to honor your spirit and your unborn child's spirit with unconditional love.

Bring in Gentle Music

Music, if gentle and in the same beat as your heartbeat (classical and spiritual), will aid in your relaxation. Methods that calm and center you will help you throughout your pregnancy and life.

Bring in a Wonderful Scent

A favorite perfume might bring loving memories that draw your consciousness to peace. These unseen molecules float through the air and interact with our senses. The sense of smell is just composed of cells that register tiny chemical substances and identify them, like vanilla or musk. At the chemical level of identification, we are registering jumps of electrons that give off waves of light, subtle energy waves.

Bring in Comfortable Clothes

Loose clothes, comfortable clothes, or no clothes should be worn during these exercises. These clothes should be white to reflect all wavelengths of color, and they should be natural. Cotton, linen, silk, or wool fibers enhance the subtle energy. They are part of nature and interact with the subtle energies of life.

The Chinese meridian system demonstrates that our bodies are streams of energy that flow out from the center of our bodies and back again. There are twelve lines that map the electrical flow through our tissue; ten represent an internal organ system, and two are centering for the entire body. When they flow unencumbered, exiting from one finger and returning through the next, these lines of energy revitalize and restore our bodies. When you go to an acupuncturist, a needle or a 1.5-volt electrical jolt is placed on one of the 950 mapped points to open and release the resistance in the tissue (resistance is saltlike deposits from tissue fluids), which moves the energy through the meridian (energy line).

Having bare hands and bare feet are natural to our bodies and enhance the energy flow. Get into a comfortable position. It is important to have your body at rest to perceive subtle energy. Scan your body with your eyes closed. Try not to feel an ache in your back or a twist in your knee. Try to be in a position where pillows and cushions support all the nooks and crannies and relieve all the aches. Quieting the physical body is as important as quieting the mental body.

Bring in a Pet

Animals seem to live on multiple levels of consciousness. If you have a pet, allow this animal spirit to move freely in your sacred space. Animals are completely, unconditionally loving. If you reflect this energy out, you will receive it back with great joy.

Bring in Water

Water refreshes. It is the lifeblood of the earth and all loving beings on it. Holy water is blessed water or ancient water from a specific area on the earth, or a holy church site, where the energies have shifted magnetically due to the bedrock deep in the ground. These waters are altered and are called structured water. The surface tension and absorption rate has changed. Dr. Marcel Vogel and Rudolf Steiner, two great scientists of the past century, have found structural changes in water that enhance life. Structured water is the scientific term for prayed upon water. This live water is what you want to feed your tissues and the newly forming cells of your unborn child.

For centuries, sacred water came from sacred springs and rivers that today are still visited by thousands to receive these healing energies.

Create your own sacred water by using springwater and saying a prayer over it, as you were taught as a child to do before meals. This helps make the intention and consciousness of God flow into your food. Ask the Holy Spirit, Christ, and God to bless your water, and then give thanks for these blessings of life.

Now, as you look around your space, the subtle energies of nature surround and enliven you. Next, cleanse and purify your energy so it will become one with the energies of life.

Enlivening the Subtle Energy of Your Spirit

The aura that surrounds your body is a field of energy. That energy is a blend of wavelengths that express themselves as your physical tissue. When there are irritating subtle energies in your field, it is very difficult to quiet your mind and identify the spiritual energy of your unborn child. Here are four ancient techniques to cleanse your subtle energy:

Prayer

We are spirit in physical form. The honoring of that spirit renews our mind, our body, and our soul. In prayer, we quietly commune with the essence of spirit. We ask humbly to this sacred energy to help and guide us on our journey through life. Our energy fields are part of this subtle energy of life. As we take a breath in with intention, we take in a nourishing breath of life that feeds our physical lungs and the flow of life energy up and down our spine.

The cleansing of our energy field occurs when we breathe in the love of God deep into our tissue. This floods our body with light and love, pushing our field outward to interact with nature. Sensitives, religious leaders, health-care providers, scientists, and dowsers have acknowledged this energy expansion with prayer for centuries. Filling your field with a consciousness of love of God is the highest energy that we can perceive; therefore, at this time, it is our highest potential to attune and cleanse our field. Breathe in the love of God, hold your breath as long as possible, allow this thought to permeate your tissues, and gently breathe out all interfering waveforms that create disharmony in your field. Give thanks for the healing you have received, and relax.

Smudging

Indigenous tribes all over the earth believed in the purification by smoke. The actual charged molecules of smoke that are visible travel through the air, breaking up congealed masses of charged particles that are invisible. The Aborigines of Australia and the North American Indians would light a dried sacred herb and cleanse you with the smoke. The smudge stick of herbs would be held about three to ten inches from the skin and swept over the entire body, just as if you were in the shower with a bar of soap.

Sweat Lodge ceremonies are steam-filled tepees or huts that purify your body and spirit, enhancing vision quests. It is an ancient water-purification technique.

Common ceremonies today are purifying with smoke and sacred herbs before the priest walks into church, during funerals around the casket and at the time of baptism.

When Christ was born, the three sacred gifts were gold, frankincense, and myrrh, gold and ceremonial smudging herbs. Gold represents kingship. Frankincense represents holiness; it is the resin of the *Boswellia thurfera* tree in Arabia. It has a star-shaped flower and a lemon fragrance. Myrrh symbolizes the suffering that is endured in a lifetime. It is a small tree, *Commiphora myrrha*, from East Africa. If the stem is cut, a few drops of myrrh will drop out and solidify. It is dark orange to brown in color.

The cleansing of your energy field renews a lightness to the body that you can feel. The process is to obtain a smudge stick (sage, sweetgrass, or cedar) or a stick of incense, or even sage from your spice cabinet (bless the herb with a prayer). Place the loose herb in a fireproof bowl, and light it, then blow it out gently so it is smoldering. If you use an incense stick, light it and use it like a wand. Start at your feet, and try to carefully, slowly pass the smoke through every inch of space around your body. If the smudge stick goes out, you must light it again, repeating the procedure until that area can be smudged without the irritating energies putting out the fire. Be very careful to never touch your body, hair, or clothes or anything flammable with the smudge stick. Be careful!

When you have completed the exercise, close your eyes, take a deep breath in sending it deep into the womb, and relax. Try to note the sensations of peace that you might feel due to this cleansing process.

Sound

Sounds bathe our bodies with subtle vibrations that pass through our tissue. Just as smoke reacts with the subtle energies of the aura, so is sound also a great purifier.

Obtain a musical instrument that creates a perfect pitch. The most accessible is a tuning fork. A crystal bowl (toning bowl) or a Tibetan bowl may also be used. If you strike the tuning fork and slowly pass it over the center of your body from your head to your toe, the same pitch should be audible throughout the passage of the energy field. The sound of the tuning fork will distort over an area that has irritating hovering waveforms. This easy experiment should be done often to cleanse these distorting waveforms from your field. If a distortion is heard, repeat passing the perfect pitch over and over through your aura. This waveform creates interference patterns with the irritation in the field and breaks up the discharge in the area, cleansing the field.

Color

Visible light makes our world come alive. We are all colors. These hues of light interact with our cells, helping to create moods. The greens of spring are physically enlivening, the blue sky soothes and calms, and the color red energizes. It is possible to feel colors in a way that allow them to penetrate your subtle energies.

Obtain a large plastic sheet of colored paper, called a gel sheet, at your local art-supply store. Gel sheets are used in the theater over lights to bathe the actress in a field of light waves. Choose a color that you love, or choose baby pink, the color of your energy field at this time. It represents unconditional love and pregnancy.

Place this gel in a window. When the sun shines through, take off your clothes and let the color bathe you with light. These gentle invisible rays cover your field with energy. Relax, breathe, and try to feel the subtle energy. These energies are subtle, and you may take as long as you like to sense the difference between the single waveform of color and the sun, which has the waveforms of all color.

Always breathe in the color with intention, deep into your tissues, and see the color bathe each organ. This will enhance this experience.

Now as you begin to have a sense of your own energy field, the energy of your space, and the energy field of your sacred objects in the room, you are now ready to feel the energy of your baby.

Everything you see and feel, the child experiences through you. The physical sensations the child evaluates are forms of vibrational energy that the child is just beginning to interpret.

Realize that the home of your child at this moment depends on you, the caretaker. How the child senses and feels begins now, not after birth.

If you experience the vibrations of energy that surround you daily, you become more conscious of life. Spirit is life, and this wonderful acknowledgment creates a baby that feels welcomed, loved, and safe.

Lesson 3
Spiritual Communication

Communication is an exchanging of ideas and information. The feelings conveyed between the parent and the unborn child are very intimate. When you are pregnant, you have the potential to send your thoughts and to commune with your unborn child, because this child is partially in the spirit world and partially in the physical. Your physical cells are one. Your fluids intermingle. Your needs can be felt. The being inside of yourself is sharing your thoughts. What greater opportunity can we have than to commune with this special soul that is being created from your own tissue? In a spiritual sense and a genetic sense, this child carries your consciousness.

When we try to reconnect with that sacred part of consciousness, we are attempting spiritual communication. At this time in your life, you are closest to the energy of the creation of consciousness. There can be no earthly value placed on this intimate experience. The consciousness of all of life is interwoven into an energy that we can choose to access every day. The ability to relate to this energy involves an awareness of a harmony with all things. This harmony allows you to commune with the subtle energy of pregnancy. You touch a level of communing with that inner soul. That soul is currently residing in your body. You can recognize and associate the intimate feelings and sensations of pregnancy with the energies of life.

When you feel, your unborn child receives information that is filtered through your thoughts and transferred into chemicals that produce emotions and actions. When your hormone levels rise (stress or joy), the child recognizes the instant chemical shifts that produce energy shifts. The pulse of life is based on these energy waves.

Life is moving fluid consciousness. This unhindered movement of consciousness creates joy.

Spiritual communication is an exchanging and interacting with subtle energies. As a mother, you become more keenly aware of these subtle energy shifts. You might call it at times a women's intuition or sixth sense; it really is the ability to recognize energy shifts that are in the spiritual energy field. Quiet time should be spent between the parent and the unborn child identifying these subtle energies that surround you both at this time. As you begin to communicate in this manner, the unborn child begins to recognize these energy shifts also. An intimate relationship begins to evolve. This involves the spiritual nature of matter. The relationship continues to grow into the birth and life journey of the parent and child, bringing a subtle energy harmony into your home. The subtle energies that the young child feels can be acknowledged and discussed by the family. A simple example of the subtle physical changes felt by the child could be described on a sunny day. You can explain it; today is sunny, and the air is fresh and clean. Feel and breathe into the uterus this alive, vibrant air and sunlight. Feel the energy, and offer its sense of joy to your child. Feel life with the child today.

This interaction and acknowledgment of the consciousness of the child on a daily basis encourages that child to interact in return. This type of subtle energy exchange has been done through the centuries between the mother and unborn child. Begin to think and feel different forms of spiritual communication, and try the techniques with patience and joy.

The different forms of spiritual communication are sacred words that attempt to describe a conscious experience that is a spiritual truth.

Spiritual communication has always existed. We have prayed for answers since our first conscious thought. Spirit resides in all of God's creations. In our prehistory, we prayed to the sun and our mother earth. It was a great evolutionary leap to perceive the concept of a consciousness of God. A Creator of our solar system, a Creator of all.

Prehistoric forms of spiritual communication are still practiced on the planet today. There is still a spiritual sense of life that tribal people connect with. Their form of communication is also trying to reach an understanding of God, the Creator of all things. Indigenous tribes have a sense of spirit that is timeless.

Spiritual communication is a voice from your soul whose source is in the mind of God. It can be a visionary dream, a meditation that brings peace, or an answered prayer. It could be a symbolic message from the Holy Spirit or an answered prayer from Christ. The Holy

Spirit is that part of consciousness that communes with the divine, lighting and guiding our path.

Shamanic Journeying

In remote areas, there are indigenous tribes that do not conform to any of the major religions of our day, yet they are in prayerful meditation with the spirit of the creator of all things. Their prayerful meditation is called shamanic journeying. This method of spiritual communication is a powerful form of ritual and prayer that is thousands of years old.

Shamanic journeying is like a guided imagery technique. A rhythmic drumming in the background quiets your conscious mind and allows your semiconscious to ask the divine a question and then search the heavens and earth for the answer. The answer comes as a vision or picture or voice.

Meditation

The yogis used meditation to quiet the mind and listen to the spirit for their answers. If you quiet the mind, the physical and the emotional bodies, then you can listen in deep prayer to the divine.

Kahuna

The Kahunas of Hawaii prayed with intention. They would breathe rhythmically the breath of life into the palms of their hands until a heavy ball of energy was formed. They would then give this as a gift to the soul of the person in need. Their prayer techniques were so many centuries old that the Christian missionaries had to try to understand how they perceived spirit before they could teach them about Christ.

Dowsing

Dowsing is a form of divining that has been used for centuries. Dowsing is a neuromuscular response to an energy shift in our environment. It is our muscular response to thoughts. This form of spiritual communication is taught by experienced professionals who have used these methods for years. The ASD (American Society of Dowsers) in Danville, Vermont, with great spiritual conscience, guided thousands of people to use these simple tools. There are dowsing societies in almost every country in the world. Historically, Moses was the first dowser, asking in prayer for God to give the tribes their needed water as they wandered in the wilderness.

Feng Shui

The Chinese use a technique called feng shui, which also has a thousand-year history.

Feng shui is another form of divining, or asking God through prayer, the correct placement for harmony of all the energies at a site. This is so honored a method of communing with the forces of nature that God created that major buildings are first energetically evaluated before the architect begins his/her designs. The Forbidden City of Beijing was created according to feng shui principles. Feng (wind) is the unmanifest forces, and shui (water) is the manifest physical environment. This form of spiritual communication is communing between the physical world and the spiritual world to create harmony so all the energies flow.

Dreams

Dreams are a form of our subconscious trying to communicate and awaken or draw thoughts into our consciousness. When you wake up and remember a dream, write it down. Keep a dream journal during pregnancy. You may ask a question to yourself before you sleep, asking for the answer in a dream. This form of spiritual communication teaches a level of trust between your mind and your spirit. You may ask the spirit of your unborn child what name would they like to be called, or is there somewhere they would like to go? Try to be open to receive communication in a variety of forms. Then try to go deep into your soul and evaluate the information you have received.

Clairvoyance, Clairaudience, and Clairsentience

Clairvoyance, *clairaudience*, and *clairsentience* are words that attempt to describe a spiritual seeing, hearing, and knowing. Many times, in prayer or meditation, we receive visions or knowledge that we follow because of our faith. These forms of spiritual communication during prayer are the faith that brings you to the truth that your unborn child is part of the spirit of God consciousness. This spirit is also in you. When you are quietly thinking about these lessons, always open your heart and ask this child to communicate with you. Honor that communication in any form, whether it is a physical kick, a dream, a vision in prayer, or a midnight craving for melon. Each time you honor and acknowledge this child, you have sent loving thoughts that commune with this child's soul. Always give thanks for the joy of both your spirits. Through the years, we have created many terms that fit many cultures but have the same meaning. Realize that God, Christ, and your Holy Spirit are with you always, and not dependent upon language or terms.

Prayer with Intention

Spiritual communication is a very personal experience. Whatever name or form you choose, the heart and soul of this communication is prayer with intention. Prayer is the act of communication from humans to the divine. You may ask for guidance, request a wish, or just express joy and thankfulness.

Honor the religious beliefs of your ancestors and the energy of centuries of their repeated prayers. Millions have tried to seek to communicate with that part of spirit that is one with its creator. A simple method is sometimes the most powerful method. Ask the Holy Spirit, say a prayer from your traditional religion, and wait and listen. Trust and wait. This simple method has been successful since the beginning of time.

Lesson 4
Spiritual Touch

Spiritual touch begins with a delicate sensing, using your fingertips. Many times it does not involve actual physical touching. When you are trying to detect a very fine subtle energy, you must use more than one sense at a time. You might interweave your feeling and smelling with touching to understand fully and on many levels what you are experiencing. When spiritual touch is described in these lessons, it is a touch experienced with your whole body. It becomes an energy interaction rather than a physical touching. It requires little practice and a keen awareness that develops over time. It is natural to feel something when you are near someone special to you. We have a closeness of family and/or friends because we are feeling love and support from these beings. On many levels, we spiritually are interacting with each other. An acknowledgement of this type of interaction with different energy forms leads us to understand it and experience it more deeply.

An example of spiritual touch could begin with a common household plant or a bouquet of flowers.

Try to relax and focus on the plant in front of you. Gently rub your hands together, as if you were washing them without soap. This increases the surface blood flow and brings a charge of your energy to the surface. First, observe the plant with your eyes open. This gives you a familiar feeling. It is a plant, it has leaves, it is in soil or water, it might have flowers, it could be a succulent or an evergreen. Now close your eyes, and gently rub your hands together again. When they feel warm and comfortable, reach forward, toward the plant. Try not to touch the plant but to feel if you can sense the plant without touching it. Spiritually see if you are near the leaf or the flower; is there a different feeling? Open your eyes and see if you were correct. Do the leaf and the flower have a different smell? You can smell the difference between the leaf and the flower and the soil. Can you sense the difference in energy with your eyes closed?

Just like people, every plant has a personality. It is the same with souls, even the souls of unborn children. You may not feel the energy the first time you try this experiment. Be patient, and know that your child feels this energy. It is a playful time between you and your child. Try this technique with your sacred rock, a bowl of water, a box of soil, or a tree. Each will have its own subtle energy. You may feel all of these as different energies, or you might feel nothing. Don't struggle with an outcome, just relax and enjoy yourself.

The feelings of love and intimacy can be felt on many levels. These exercises bring you closer to the subtle energies of life. Life, in all forms, is a creation of God. The lessons in this book demonstrate approaches to the subtle energy of life. Life is energy. Your ability to interact and observe these energies creates a more intimate relationship with spirit.

Lesson 5
The Spiritual Intimacy of Motherhood

For this moment in time, open your heart to truly welcome this incoming soul that has allowed you to experience the physical changes of motherhood. Open your heart to the intermingling energy of your soul and your unborn child's soul. Rest and relax in love.

The energy surrounding your body is changing. Women often have a beautiful soft pink aura of unconditional love; this is the color of the energy of mothering and nurturing. This energy surrounds the child and blankets the mother in a protective envelope. This shifting energy field forms a large bubble of protection that extends to the knees and engulfs the uterus. This wave of pulsating life energy is constantly monitoring all vibrations that affect the child or the mother. This field stops any irregular inharmonious vibrations from entering the womb. This field is so dense that it is easily detectable.

Place your right hand over the uterus area, approximately four to six inches above the body. Start first with the right hand and then repeat with the left. Scan the energy field to feel first an envelope of heat. It will feel like a warm barrier of protective energy. The hand will sense a gentle resistance or thickness as you move toward the body surface, a feeling of a bumper that protects and surrounds the uterus. If you approach from the knee area up, toward the mid-thigh very slowly and with conscious intention, you will feel a very firm resistance at about mid-thigh. You can increase your sensitivity to this by practicing. Physical pressure and energy field resistance is a feeling as if your fingers were pushing through thick fudge. You might feel hot pockets or cold spots in the energy field. Remember there are constant shifts of energy that must occur to keep the body in equilibrium.

Moving in a direction of true spiritual intimacy is acknowledging and respecting the spiritual energy that surrounds and envelopes each of us. To acknowledge the sacredness of ourselves, we must also acknowledge the sacredness of each other. Always be observant of your feelings and thoughts. Consider your worthiness and the worthiness of others. Spiritual intimacy is seeing with your soul rather than your eyes.

If you are not pregnant yet but wish to begin exercises to develop a spiritual intimacy, you might do this during intercourse. Intercourse brings forth a subtle body change in the mother. You might even have a spiritual intuition that you have conceived a child. This type of shift in the energy field comes at the moment of conception. The energy of life rises like a wave, traveling up the spine and bathing the brain in fluid. This intertwining energy (Kundalini) of life and breath is the symbol of the medical profession, the caduceus (a staff with two snakes curled around it and with two wings at the top). This is also called the staff of Hermes.

When you begin feeling these subtle energy changes, you can detect them much easier. This sensing in the energy field is very subtle. Try over and over again until you feel something with your hands. You may feel more with your left hand than with your right. Your feeling might come from a knowing rather than a feeling of heat or density. Each person has developed their senses in a way appropriate to their environment. One way is not better than another. It may take many different lessons to find the messages that are sent through your subtle energy field. Always have patience.

Acknowledge, love, and honor your senses. Trust that your spirit will direct you.

In many cultures, the ancient belief was that the father's sperm was the only nutrient the unborn child received. This energy exchange was believed to be crucial to the child's survival. Both parents were involved in the growth of the child. Both male and female energy was required to produce a healthy child. Today we know the importance of the diet and health of the mother. The question is, on a subtle energy basis, does the father's energy enhance the subtle energy of the child? Because the child receives half of its genetic material from a male energy, it can only enhance the child to be bathed in that energy from time to time. Therefore, the spiritual energy and intimacy of motherhood should be concerned with, if it is possible, a deep involvement of the father.

Other children in the family or grandparents can be taught to sense the energy around the child. This will have them interact with the child so the unborn child will recognize their individual voices and energy patterns. This will bring a greater spiritual intimacy into the family. It will bring the energy of the family to the unborn child and give them a feeling of welcome. Begin slowly; rest and relax in love.

Lesson 6
Divine Visualization

To begin this or any visualization, try to relax and be aware of your body. Focus on your intention. To focus on your intention, you should clear your mind. Close your eyes, and breathe deep breaths, as if these breaths could reach every cell and the deepest parts of your soul. With your eyes closed, see a blank movie screen in front of you. Pretend you are in a darkened theater, awaiting the show. Your mind should feel open and relaxed. Relaxation begins to occur with a quieting of the mind and a few deep breaths. Breathe deeply into your body, feeling your chest and abdomen fill with fresh, sweet air. Breathe rhythmically, and send the life-giving breath to all your tissue. Breathe deeply into your womb. If you would like, you may read the visualization that is on the next page "A Gift from God" out loud so the child will feel the vibrations of your voice. You may read it to yourself and send the sense of calm to the child upon completion, or you may read and think of each intention as you read, mentally sending the calming thoughts to your child.

Visualizing is a mental body task. This means that your physical and emotional bodies must be at peace. To create a peaceful physical body, you should be wearing soft, comfortable clothes and be surrounded by things of nature: plants and flowers, a bowl of clean, clear water from a nearby brook or ocean, a box of fresh soil you can place your feet in. Feeling all these earthly energies will bring a feeling of peace to your meditation. Soft candlelight or sunlight is preferred over electric light because you need the qualities of full-spectrum light. Your emotional body should be nurtured by surroundings of love and joy. A photograph of loved ones or a token memory of someone who has passed away brings feelings of loving moments. These mementos help to create your sacred space. When you feel quite calm and nurtured by your special space, you are ready to begin. Slowly read with intention the following:

A Gift from God

I bless my body. It is the temple of God. To my physical body, I ask the Holy Spirit to send energy and vigor. To my emotional body, I ask the Holy Spirit to send joy and love. I bathe my emotional body with warm calm waters. To my mental body, I ask the Holy Spirit to send peace and tranquility. My spiritual body receives harmony and spiritual love always. These are all different vibration levels of the same substance: pure spiritual energy. Every cell in my body is relaxed and in harmony with God. Each organ in my body is in harmony. My subtle energy, harmony, and wholeness expresses my spiritual self.

I bless my body and give thanks for it. It is the living, breathing individualization of God. The essence of spirit circulates my blood, controls my life functions, and cares for every cell in my body. The essence of spirit directs the growth of my child. The kingdom of God dwells within me. The spirit of my healthy and joyful child dwells within me. I am thankful for the loving care of us both. I can feel every cell in my child's body being activated by the light and love of God. My child is forming organs and tissue that are in harmony with the will of God, creating a loving wholeness that is God, expressing itself as a new being. I bless this new being and give thanks for its expression of joy. I thank thee, Father, for thy loving care of my unborn child.

Amen.

And so it is.

Sit back and relax for a moment, and breathe deeply into your uterus. With a mindful prayer, send inward the love of God. Breathe into the uterus the love you offer your child. Gently stroke your tummy with a soft clockwise motion as you breathe into the womb.

My child is a gift from God, and I thank you for this wonderful experience.

Lesson 7
Myth and Magic

In all myth, there is a thread of truth. In our inability to explain spiritual events, we create stories that symbolically describe the subtle energy of spirit. We can feel that subtle floating energy of spirit as we watch birds soar. We can feel it as we listen to their sweet chirping.

Acknowledging other forms of God's creation brings us onto a deeper level of our own creation. This allows us the freedom of sensing our connectedness to all of God's life-forms.

Our old wives' tales talked about as folklore today were based on the spiritual belief of that moment in time. They live on as myth and legend until we evolve into a greater understanding of ourselves. Myths are stories that weave a tale of mystery and supernatural into the commonplace. Our spirit originates in the sacred space of the unmanifest. A place where there is no physical form. A sacred space far away in the heavens, where existence is only known to God consciousness. Our body is of the earth. Those same molecules that are in our oceans, rocks, and soils are creating our tissue fluids, bones, and organs. To create our existence, spirit and physical form must blend. Myths touch our hearts with a closeness to the mysteries of life. They create a magical world where everything is explained in terms that anyone can understand.

On earth, descriptions of the unmanifest are limited. We have attempted to describe the realm of spirit as the heavens or the sky. Throughout history, birds have represented the free-flowing spiritual essence of that unknown realm of unmanifest. The sense that the spirit of the unborn child would float through the sky, being carried by a stork, is ancient and in many cultures. In the blending of myth and magic, our souls originate from the skies, and our bodies are of the earth. The legend of the stork is just such a mystery.

Since time eternal, birds have had a direct involvement with birthing and pregnancy. Most cultures believed the spirit of the unborn child would be delivered by a bird.

To feel the myth and magic of these feathered beings, we will attempt to spiritually commune with them. During this exercise, remember you are looking into the soul of these gentle beings. If it is possible, hold a feather, close your eyes, and feel the energy of flight. These magical creatures are truly one with the skies. God watches over them.

In Celtic folklore, pregnancy was directly associated with the myth of the stork. These storks lived in remote swamps or ponds with the souls of unborn children. The birds would gather the spirit children and bring them to people's homes. They believed that children were "spirit children" having a direct connection to spirit until birth, when their connection was earthly for a few short years of life. The belief was that if a stork flew above the house, the women of the house could be impregnated by it. Some husbands built nests on their roofs to attract storks and have many children. They fed the storks with sugar placed on their roofs and windowsills.

These myths are somewhere deep in our subconscious and play a subtle energy role during critical periods of our lives. You may love watching birds or hearing their sweet song. The fact that birds have been related to pregnancy and birth for so many centuries brings us at this time an opportunity to reacknowledge their sacredness. Be grateful for their loving existence, and watch their magical spirit.

A Magical Spirit Watch

Sometime during the day, early sunrise is the most peaceful. Go outside into the fresh air. Bring a handful of fresh seeds and nuts. Relax under the nearest quiet tree. If this is not possible, use the bird feeder you have placed in your window. When a bird arrives, consider it an ancient blessing for your unborn child. The purpose is to allow nature to commune with you and your unborn child. Ask the spirit of the tree if you may quietly rest there (considering that it is the home to many animals, birds, and insects). Ask the neighboring birds in silent meditation that they bless your new God-sent spirit child. For this blessing, offer them some seeds and nuts, thanking them graciously for their presence and song and the joy they bring to all the beings of earth. Feel the delicate nature of these tiny creatures, and gently stroke your unborn child. Feel the delicate nature of this special tiny unborn child.

Observing birds in flight brings a better understanding of the subtle energy flows of the earth. Birds soar along air currents, but how do they know migration patterns? Birds have a small quantity of magnetite, a naturally occurring magnetic ore in their brain. This ore has been related to their ability to travel great distances following the subtle magnetic flows of the earth. It is believed that you also have a tiny quantity of this type of ore in your nose. Could you use this to detect subtle energy shifts? When we lived closer to nature, we lived by the ebb and flow of the tides and the energies of the moon cycles. We had a greater respect for these subtle energies. The ability to detect energy shifts in the landscape was rewarded as a place of honor in the community. We marked these energy shifts as sacred sites. England has ancient roads that follow energy ley lines, still described today as fairy paths and sacred sites. Notice the energy of these tiny birds that still live as one with nature. Notice how they all move together following the wind currents, creating a beautiful dance. As you observe your landscape, try to sense an energy shift as the birds might sense it, or a possible sacred site.

Wait and watch these tiny creatures; they are very friendly and gentle. They will visit you every day if you feed them. If you feed them at the same time of the day, they will be waiting to greet you.

When you are ready, thank again the tree and the birds and the spirit of your unborn child. Offer your blessings back to everyone, and go in peace.

Place a bird feeder in your window or yard at this special time in your life. Bring the energy and song of the bird to your unborn child. As you observe these tiny beings of joy and light, try to sense the delicate nature of their existence. It is very much like the existence of your tiny unborn child. You are nurturing and caring for your child, this special spirit that you bring into this world.

What Is Sacred?

Lesson 8
The Sacred Womb: The Sacred Body

Sacredness is a consciousness of wonder and grace that can be imparted to your unborn child. It is an energy or a sense of knowing that something very special, very unearthly is being experienced. When you acknowledge sacredness in an event, the experience and awareness is heightened. You begin to feel the consciousness of wonder and unconditional love. To begin feeling the sacredness of bringing forth a new soul into existence, you should feel the sacredness of your own body.

A comfortable place to begin would be to honor the sacredness of your womb. This energy will permeate from your physical body into your environment. Your womb is sacred space. This space allows the spiritual energy of God to enter and create a wonderful loving being—your child. Communicating the sacredness of this creation can be achieved on many levels.

Visualizing the Sacred Womb

Relax and sit in a warm comfortable area of your home, or the sacred space of peace you have created. Try to surround yourself with peace and quiet. For a few moments, you and your unborn baby will travel through time, exploring the sacred womb and the sacredness of motherhood. This sacredness has been expressed many ways. It has been expressed in all races and religions. The loving description commonly used is the *female goddess*. In you, there is a female goddess; you are symbolic of all women throughout history.

The most ancient is Isis, queen of heaven. She is described as the symbolic female who created the sun and gave birth to all living things. Close your eyes, and feel the warmth and energy of life that the sun brings forth. Feel it shining on your womb, energizing your baby. Feel its soft warmth bring forth life. The sun nurtures the plants and animals on earth as a mother nurtures her child. Feel your child receiving this energy, as does all life on earth. Be thankful for this part of our existence that creates warmth and light, bathing all living things with wavelengths of light. In Hebrew the goddess is Iso, and in Scandinavian or Gothic, she is pronounced *Isa*. *Isa* translates as "ice," which is water in its quiet crystallized state. Water has many forms. Water, in any form, is sacred to life. Water is the basic builder of life. We are created floating in the warm secure waters of the womb, and our bodies are 90 percent water. Many cultures honor the gift of water. If you live in a northern region, you would understand the Scandinavian myth.

Wherever you are, you can begin to have a feel for water in a new way. Close your eyes and relax. See your unborn child floating in the sacred warm waters of the womb. Bathed and protected in its sacred space. Think of how all life on earth depends upon water. We are a water planet. Our moon creates our ocean tides on earth, and also our female monthly cycles that create an ebb and flow of our fertility. Envision how the sacred energy of water is in all our tissues, harmonizing our bodies, creating oneness with all animals, plants, birds, and ocean and land creatures. Imagine that the ancient goddess was blessed for all this. Imagine that you are symbolically now filled with the sacred energy of water that bathes your child. Softly stroke your sacred womb, acknowledging that small angel that you carry. This dance of creation is everywhere.

In astrology, the Virgo constellation represents the universal mother. Tonight spend a moment looking up at the stars, knowing that you are a symbolic universal mother. Throughout history, you have been a sacred symbol of life. Feel the distant connections you have with the heavens. Speaking softly to your unborn child, acknowledge his/her journey from those heavenly realms into your womb, and welcome this child as a part of your family and your life. The earth, the waters, and the stars all welcome this child.

In Christianity we can compare the Virgin Mary, to theory, of this ancient goddess. She was a virgin and gave birth to Jesus the Savior. Breathe deeply into your womb, the love of God. Think and feel the love all religions have for the sacredness of motherhood. Breathing in the love of God into your womb permeates your cells with a consciousness of unconditional love and peace. As you breathe the breath of life with intention, you renew spiritual energy into your womb. You are blessed to experience such sacredness. Give thanks to God, and be aware of the sacredness of your womb and of this joyful process. This process occurs with just intention. Your intentions of peace, unconditional love, and wonder will, on many subtle energy levels, reach the spirit of your child. With intention, you have spiritually communicated your love into your womb. Give thanks for your ability to be consciously pregnant.

After you have visualized the sacred space of your womb, you can now feel how the earth creates sacred space. If you can feel the sacredness of the creation of life, can you now feel and sense it all around you?

Lesson 9
Sacred Waters

Sacred physical space is an area of special unseen subtle energies. It is a holy place, a place of communion with God, of altered consciousness. Your womb is sacred space. The subtle energy of shape, form, and creation is the energy of sacred space. As you journey through your pregnancy, you will feel the creation of life inside of you. To experience this energy outside of you, feel the earth's sacred space. With the help of earth energies, this connection becomes easier. When we search to understand the earth's sacred space, we find a closer intimate relationship with our sacred space. One method is the experience one can have with sacred sites.

Sacred sites are areas on the earth surface that contain unusually high energy emanating from them. This is a subtle electromagnetic energy. This subtle electromagnetic energy, measurable in science, can be felt by many and is not any more sacred than anything

God has created, but in ancient times, these sites were noted as unusual. Nature religions have always acknowledged these earth energies and marked them. Ancient churches were built on these special sites. Many sites have life-giving water that the ancients needed for existence. Springs, wells, and the birthplaces of rivers are sacred areas. These areas are where the earth gives forth the gift of its lifeblood—water.

Just as the blood runs through your arteries, creating life, so does the earth have water that runs through its arteries deep into its tissue. Water is the lifeblood of the earth. This is an ancient truth. Springs and wells have a special earth energy that was considered their spirit.

A gift was always given to the spirit of the well in gratitude for the healing life-giving waters and to ensure its continuance. Today this tradition is still practiced by tossing coins into wishing wells or pools of water. This is one of our superstitions. A superstition, by definition, is something that "stands over" from a previous time.

Sacred Water

Your unborn child is floating gently in a pool of life-giving water. To feel the gentle relaxation of this life-giving pool, fill the bathtub with warm water. Place a candle in the sink and light it so the light is diffused as if you are in a womb. Then offer a gift to the water. This gift is a gift of thanks for the many blessings you receive from the water. Your gift must mean something special to you. If you have a special perfume, place a few drops into the water. If your favorite herb is rosemary or thyme, place a teaspoon of that into the water. If you have a special rock or quartz crystal, place that into the water. With each special gift, you share a part of yourself, infusing your energy and loving thoughts and prayers into the water. Then, making sure the water temperature is comfortable to you, slowly submerge yourself in all these special energies. Float gently with your unborn child. Involve the father in this process if you are near a lake. Feel the molecules of water gently rolling and moving over your body, imparting this energy of movement to your senses. Freely floating in water is the same as the sensations your baby is feeling. The baby feels supported, floating, free of body weight and filled only with consciousness. Relax and massage your abdomen. Close your eyes, and feel the ancient healing energies of water. Feel its sacredness.

Lesson 10
Divining the Aura of the Unborn Child

There is a field of energy that surrounds every living thing. It is called an aura, and it reflects the physical, emotional, mental, and spiritual energy of that being. Historically, it was the domain of mystics, monks, and spiritual religious leaders. Sensing this sacred energy of the aura, the unmanifest energy of life, can be experienced using a technique called dowsing. Dowsing, or divining, is an ancient term that describes the interaction we can observe and experience with this special field of life-force energy.

Divining sites to detect energy shifts has been practiced since the beginning of time. Moses is recorded as having used a rod to discover water, and the solar deity Mithras divined water with a bow and arrow. Dowsers today find their rods respond to lines of energy sometimes called geodetic patterns. The dowser can detect a special pattern of energy (earth energy) that has a relationship to the electromagnetic field of the earth at that location that was there before the sacred site was constructed. The pattern must have been previously identified by a geomancer, a priest, a member of the arcane brotherhood, a "wise" man or woman, or even an animal. Animals are drawn to energetically "healthy" sites. The word *health* or *heal* in Northern Middle English means "to make sound." One method of detecting the subtle energies and emanations around us is to dowse. Feeling and sensing these energies brings us closer to an intimate knowledge of the subtle energies of our unborn child. Everyone can learn how to dowse. Practice is all that is required. Dowsing is an attempt to sense an electromagnetic field. Animals have the ability to detect these forces of nature. We have ignored this ability because it is not used commonly in our daily lives.

Dowsing is a way of feeling and intuiting an answer. Divining is a relationship between you and your sense of energy. A form of divining occurs daily with your prayers; it is intimate intention. It is a very personal experience that adds quality to your life. In biblical days, Aaron, Moses's brother, utilized the breastplate to ask the divine a yes-or-no question for the Hebrews.

This ancient form of prayer has evolved into our current methods of prayer, taught in churches and temples.

Using a tool to sense the energies of the womb has been done since the time of the ancients. This tool is a geometric form that interacts on a subtle energy shift, detecting an energy change. It is very similar in theory to a thermometer that reads a change in temperature. This is reacting to a change in subtle energy.

A simple method is to create a dowsing rod. This is an instrument used to learn dowsing. This rod will move in response to a subtle neuromuscular reflex in your body. This demonstration will show you how your body has a subtle energy response. Make a rod for everyone in your family. Begin by dowsing the energy field of your baby. The energy field of your unborn child is sometimes called an aura. Aura photography was first researched by Nikola Tesla (1890s). The Soviet Union included aura photography in the psychic research it conducted in the 1960s. In 1975, the University of California at Los Angeles was able to measure auras with great accuracy. McGill University, in the 1980s, researched these subtle body responses. Today, research continues to unveil the interactions we have at very subtle energy levels.

An introduction to the existence of the living field of energies is described and demonstrated in the following exercise. These rods are in a mathematical relationship to the Fibonacci series and the golden rectangle theory.

Making Angle Rods

Lesson 10 - Chart 1

Making Angle Rods- Obtain a coat hanger-
Cut on Lines-

Bend back to 90 degrees-

Cover the ends with tape-

A sleeve is best to cover the handle, allowing the rod to swing freely Empty spools of thread or a thin piece of tubing from the hardware store works great.

A simple dowsing rod is a bent wire. Coat hangers are cut in the shape described.. These simple directions help you with the basic structure. The rod is shaped with a ninety-degree angle. Cover all rough edges to protect you when holding your rods. These rods should not touch the body. A sleeve is best used to cover the handle, allowing the rod to swing freely. Empty spools of thread or a thin piece of tubing from the hardware store work great.

Practice

The goal is to hold the rods as steady as possible in a horizontal plane to your arm. Try not to tilt your arm or wrist upward of downward. Hold the rods out in front of you. Relax your mind, and set your intention: "I am going to dowse the physical energy fields of the body." This subtle energy can be detected six to eight inches out from the body. As you walk toward the person, the rods should begin to waver very slowly. At about six inches from the body, your rods will swing outward, pushed by the subtle energy that surrounds the body. Never struggle to try and get a response. The response occurs when you are at complete peace, not expecting or creating an outcome. Try it with all your family members. Some will be natural dowsers, and it will occur easily. Others may have to repeat the experiment until they are totally relaxed. Repeat this experiment.

Now dowse the physical energy of the unborn child. An incredible change occurs. A large energy bubble surrounds the baby, protecting and blanketing this sacred womb. The auric egg extends usually up to twenty or thirty inches out from the womb. The rest of the mother's body's physical energy field remain at six to eight inches out. Acknowledge the sacredness of this special subtle energy that protects our unborn children. It is an energy of creation and an energy of God. Dr. Harold Burr at Yale University discovered this energy around life in the 1950s and described it as a life energy field. Try to feel this gentle life force.

Lesson 11
A Sacred Path: Labyrinths

There are many forms of sacred space. The labyrinth is a form of sacred geometry that creates the energy of sacred space. The wisdom of the ancients is embodied in all that they construct. Temples and churches were intended to act as the physical expression of a secret wisdom. They were the symbolic manifestation of the mysteries in architectural form. Before the age of actual church structures, the ancients created sacred patterns and mazes on the earth. In many of our ancient churches, there are labyrinth structures inside the church and on church grounds. These structures are symbolic walking prayerful paths.

Labyrinths are patterns. These patterns are traced upon anything: paper, fabric, the ground, or your floor in your home. Their patterns symbolize fixed paths that meander back and forth, moving from an external world to an internal world.

When we place ourselves in a sacred mathematical shape, that shape shifts our energies. The labyrinth is an ancient shape, and as we move through it physically, our energies interact with the shape. This can be seen with a common string. If it is cut in mathematical relationships of sacred geometry and then pulled taut, it becomes a musical instrument when interacted with, creating a guitar.

The spiraling patterns of a simple labyrinth wind us into a center point and back out again, like a maze. This method of walking the sacred structure enhances spiritual communication and prayer between yourself and your spiritual essence.

Sacred space is a blessing. It connects your consciousness to the consciousness of God. It doesn't have to be a great cathedral or mosque; it is the deep intention of the seeker of spiritual communication that is important.

In the Muslim religion, they have portable prayer rugs. The design of the rug replicates the sacred geometry of the mosque. In nomadic societies, a religious person needed a traveling sacred space. The Tuareg (nomadic tribe) trace an exact outline of a mosque in the sand and step inside to pray if they did not have a prayer rug. Our creation of sacred space places our intentions on God consciousness.

Most civilizations have a mystical connection to sacred space and labyrinths. A few turf labyrinths from the Bronze Age still exist today in England. Labyrinths are found in Egyptian buildings. The Crete labyrinth, describing the sacred mythology of the Minotaur and Theseus, can still be walked today. South America has huge walking labyrinths that are called Nascar animals; these can only be seen in total from the sky.

In Chartres Cathedral (France), over the doorway, sunlight pours through the stained-glass window onto the floor, spreading light on the labyrinth walk. On the solstice (earth's seasonal energy changes), the alignment of the geometry of light and sacred math unite to create an especially holy and interactive path.

All structures had a deeply spiritual connection to the symbolic communication with your spirit. The entrance to all sacred sites is guarded by pillars or spirits. Remnants of this tradition are the carving of small heads in the Romanesque and Gothic periods of church architecture.

Looking toward the door, there is a male head on the left and a female head on the right, the position of the bridegroom and bride at Christian weddings. In our ancient history these forms were important, but now we can look at these historical images as ancient ways that the church could communicate sacredness to its community. Today you can walk this ancient path and say a simple prayer of thanks. It is very peaceful to experience a walking prayer, whether you walk a labyrinth and pray or walk to the grocery store and pray. Movement and prayer create a sacred space for you and your child.

How to Approach the Labyrinth

Traveling through the labyrinth represents a mystical journey through the twists and turns of life, to the center. In the center, you ask your sacred question then wait quietly in the center to wait in silent prayer, feeling your yes-or-no answer, waiting quietly to determine if you sense an answer. Then follow the path out again. Your answer is a gift from your soul as it travels to other levels of consciousness during the labyrinth journey.

Before entering the labyrinth, ask a question, enter, follow the path to the center, wait for your answer, and then follow the path out again. As you enter your labyrinth, it is a special geometry that is demonstrating sacred space. If you cannot create a labyrinth, go to church, say a simple prayer before walking up to the altar. During this sacred walk, observe how you feel when you consciously enter the sacred space of your church.

Creating Your Labyrinth

Lesson 11- Chart 1

A Labyrinth-

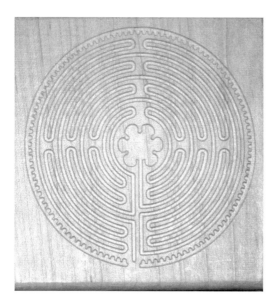

Celebrate your pregnancy. Create a labyrinth, and trace it as a morning meditation. Trace the diagram using a pencil, or create a larger labyrinth. If you make it large enough (four yards of fabric), it can be placed on the floor, and you can walk the labyrinth. Before entering, set your intention on communication, greetings, and welcome for your unborn child. Slowly follow the path out. Enjoy it for the journey inward and the meditation in the center and the journey outward. You can follow the path on this chart with your index finger.

Music and Sound

Lesson 12
Myth and Magic: Words into Sounds

Legends have always told of the divine origin of music. In mythology, music was a gift from supernatural beings. In the Jewish and Christian religious philosophy, all of the universe was created by one sound, and its unfolding and transformation creates all that exists. The Bible states that in the beginning was the word, which means a sound occurred before creation.

The singing of Psalms was believed to have healing power. Each psalm was chanted to heal a different ailment. There is a very magical power to words and tones.

The words we speak emit a sound, which corresponds to a certain color and a specific physical shape. Everything pulsates to its own tone. Ernst Chladni (1787), the father of cymatics (the study of the effects of sound waves on physical matter), realized when we speak, we create form. When the syllables of the ancient language of Sanskrit and Hebrew were pronounced (spoken into a microphone attached to a metal plate with sand on top), the sand took the form of the written symbols of those sounds.

When a soul incarnates, it sends a vibration that sounds a tone throughout the universe. Each one of us has a theme song, frequency that is created by the words we call ourselves. Each name has a melody.

Numerology describes an energy to each number. An example of this is the fact that 0 was not considered a number for centuries because it denoted nothing. It was the belief that God was everywhere and assigned to the number 1, so to use 0 was against religious philosophy. The numbers 1–9 fit neatly into all philosophy. The alphabet, if you were to divide it evenly among the numbers 1–9, you would obtain the list below. The center of our musical system is the middle C. We all have a harmony to notes above and below middle C. That is why the chart begins with 1 as middle C.

To determine the melody of your name and the name you are choosing for your unborn child, you may use the following:

Lesson 12 - Chart 1

Number	Letter	Musical Note
1	AJS	Middle C
2	BKT	D
3	CLU	E
4	DMV	F
5	ENW	G
6	FOX	A
7	GPY	B
8	HQZ	High C
9	IR	High D

C	A	T	H	Y	- Name
E	Mid C	D	High C	B	- Musical Note

A	P	R	I	L	5 -Date
Mid C	B	High D	High D	E	G - Musical Note

I	L	O	V	E	Y	O	U	- Sentence
High D	E	A	F	G	B	A	E	- Musical Note

W	A	T	E	R	- Word
G	Mid C	D	G	High D	- Musical Note

Transfer your name and the chosen name of your unborn child into a musical melody, as I have demonstrated in chart 1. You can also feel the sound of the birthdate. You can transform musically the week of the due date into a welcoming song for your baby.

Your life song has a wonderful soothing effect on stress and tension. It brings you to a harmonious state of inner peace.

Commune with your unborn child musically by gently and softly singing the birth name you have chosen. Try to feel the baby floating on the waves of this beautiful melody. You can play these notes on a small piano or other musical instrument. You can meditate on each tone to feel the subtle energy of your unborn child.

Feel the divine energy of sound. Closing your eyes, see with your mind's eye. Watch for colors to appear. A state of inner peace brings waves of soft hues.

This song can be utilized to soothe you and your unborn child throughout pregnancy. Feel yourself attuned to the music. Frequent repetition is a wonderful way to lift the consciousness above the difficulties of daily living. Create a sacred space that is filled with the melody of you and your unborn child. Offer thanks for the creation of music and the beauty it has brought the world.

The Sound of Water

Your child is floating in a frequency of water that cradles and nurtures this new life. This sound is healing and loving to your child. Create the sound of water, and tone it to surround your child in a loving melody of fluid and gentle sounds. You can also have family members sing "I love you" while lightly massaging the baby.

Combine all the messages offered by each family member to create a special song of welcome for your unborn child. Create a beautiful prayer of joy to sing to your child.

Lesson 13
Musical Notes and Organ Growth

In many ways, music expresses all aspects of our lives. It has a feminine and masculine nature to it. In Chinese philosophy, flats are feminine and represent matter and physical form. Sharps are masculine and represent spirit energy. Also similar to this is the Native American philosophy that believes in two great forces. The forces of Mother Earth (form and nature) and Father Sky (spirit) join together to create balance and harmony. In Chinese philosophy, the female is called yin, which is dark and passive, and the male is called yang, being light and active.

In order to balance these great forces of nature, we are a reflection of yin and yang in every cell of our body. It is a beautiful ancient Chinese description of the energy of God that permeates all that is. Yin-yang can be used to describe the ocean waves, the movement of the planets, and the growth of your unborn child.

When you feel the creation of your unborn child, it is as if you are hearing a wave of passive and active notes expressing themselves as physical tissue.

The Chinese have known for centuries that the energy flows of the body create musical harmony. Each organ is formed by a vibration or musical note. Each organ has a tone or sound that creates it. When all organs are formed, a musical scale is created, and the being is whole. Chinese philosophy is thousands of years old. There are six yin organs that have a corresponding keynote. In the study of acupuncture and meridian therapy, most books describe the interconnectedness of our organs with sounds. The diagnosis is not based on blood tests, like our society does, but on the areas of irregular skin tone, the change of energy in the twelve pulses of the wrist, and the sounds the patient repeatedly creates. Do they sing all their sentences, are they always shouting, or do they have missing sounds, like we have missing vitamins? Meridian therapy also describes the yearly seasons as an ebb and flow of energy in and out of specific organs. The chart below lists the tone that creates harmony in the corresponding organ. There are yin and yang (expansive and contractive) organs.

Organs

There are six yin organs that have a corresponding musical key note: C—spleen (low C), D—lung (low D), E—liver (low E), F—heart and pericardium, and A—kidney. There are six yang organs that have a corresponding musical key note: G—small intestine, A—bladder, C—stomach, D—large intestine, E—gallbladder, and G—small intestine (high G).

Musical Meditation

Sit down in a comfortable position. Relax and take a few deep breaths to relax your diaphragm. When you are relaxed, begin toning and sending the beautiful notes and love to your unborn child. Rest and relax, trying to feel the body responses to the musical sounds. The organs God has created contain the sounds of life. These musical notes represent all the sounds of life. Our bodies are a symphony of subtle energy sounds. Even if you have very little knowledge of music, a beautiful, loving song from church or a favorite song from your childhood, or a prayer or psalm, will bathe your unborn child in a mother's love. Your baby hears these vibrations and their gentle loving thoughts as you sing.

Lesson 14
Emotions and Tones

There are many spiritual levels in our God-created body. These levels can be described as the emotional, mental, and spiritual subtle energy levels. The emotional and mental levels have been researched thousands of years ago. For centuries, the Chinese have labeled each point in the acupuncture system with subtle meanings. In today's meditation, try to think about each organ, and send God's love and happiness to each organ. A musical visualization can bring you and your unborn child into the sacred space of creation through music, thoughts, emotions, and sound.

Lesson 14 - Chart 1

Organ	Emotion
Liver	Happiness, Unhappiness, Anger
Gall Bladder	Gall, Bitterness, Rage
Heart	Love, Relationships, Forgiveness
Small Intestine	Joy
Spleen	Anger, Obsession
Stomach	Contentment, Tranquility, Sympathy, Disappointment, Disgust
Lung	Grief, Tolerance, Intolerance
Large Intestine	Self-Worth, Guilt, Letting Go of the Past
Kidney	Security in the Future, Children, Fear
Bladder	Anxiety, Peace, Harmony, Impatience
Reproduction/Circulation	Nurturing, Mothering, Heart Tightness
Pancreas	Sweetness of Life, Sympathy, Obsessions

Musical Meditation

As spirit comes into form, the light of God creates physical tissue. This spiritual vibration slows until it becomes physical matter. Each vibration has a corresponding tone to it. As your child grows, it requires all the tones of physical matter to create this miraculous human body.

Today's exercise combines toning a special note with the visualization of the organ that corresponds to that note. If you have a musical instrument, or even a child's piano (with notes marked), this will help you during this exercise. Visualize the positive emotions that create the sound of each organ, along with their physical function and the tone that speaks their name. Remember, all organs are forming in the first two weeks of pregnancy and are constantly growing; all but the lungs will begin function before birth.

Yin Organs

Feel the feminine nature to these yin organs; they are organs of the earth, dark and passive.

Spleen

While toning a low C and middle C in repetition, visualize physical energy coming into your unborn child and helping to harmonize the cells that are creating the spleen. The spleen is an organ that cleanses the blood. Ask for the release of all anger and obsession from the spleen of the unborn child so that she/he may live a joyful, loving life. Relax and listen to the sound of spleen.

Lung

While toning a low D, visualize subtle spiritual energy flowing into your unborn child. This energy is helping to harmonize the creation of the cells of the lung. The lungs are called the organs of tolerance and intolerance, and they allow you to breathe in the breath of life. Take a deep breath in, and see this breath of life flow into the lungs of your unborn child. Ask for a balance to occur between tolerance and intolerance. This balance creates the pure tone of unconditional love. Feel your child is bathed in this love at this very moment. Relax and listen to the sound of the lung.

Liver

While toning a low E, visualize the flowing energy of happiness into your unborn child. This happy energy is harmonizing the creation of the cells of the liver. The liver is called the organ of happiness and unhappiness. The liver is a grand detoxifying organ and the creator of magical enzymes to help all the bodily functions. The liver comes from the words *to live*. Take a deep breath in, and see the life and happiness flow into the liver of your unborn child. Create happiness, and send this subtle energy to your unborn child. Relax and listen to the sound of the liver.

Heart

While toning a note of F, visualize the subtle unconditional love you have for your unborn child. This unconditional love permeates the heart of your child and creates an unearthly peace and harmony. As the heart pumps, the blood is creating paths, vessels, arteries, and veins until all the areas of the unborn child are united. All organs touch each other through blood flow. The blood is considered the most sacred of all tissue. Visualize the energy of love harmonizing the creation of the cells of the heart. Take a deep breath in, and see the kindness, love, and forgiveness this unborn soul offers you. Accept graciously the love of this special relationship. Relax and listen to the sound of the heart.

Kidney

While toning a note of A, visualize the energy of security flowing into your unborn child. This energy is helping to harmonize the creation of the cells of the kidneys. The kidneys regulate and cleanse the fluids of the body.

Take a deep breath in and see the unborn child safe and secure, now and in the future. Relax and listen to the sound of the kidneys.

Yang Organs

Feel the masculine spiritual energy of these yang organs. These are organs of the sky. They are light and active.

Small Intestine

While toning a G and then a high G in repetition, visualize the subtle energy of joy coming into your energy field. This joyful energy is helping to create the organ of the small intestine. The small intestine digests and absorbs the food you eat and the fluids you drink. Bring into the unborn child the nurturing energy of life. This is the ability to transform food into life energy, strength, love, and joy. Relax and listen to the sound of the small intestine.

Bladder

While toning an A, visualize the subtle energy of peace, patience, and harmony coming into your unborn child. This peaceful energy is creating the organ of the bladder. The bladder holds the liquids of the body in storage before releasing them. Relax and listen to the sound of the bladder.

Stomach

While toning the note of C, visualize the emotion of contentment and tranquility flowing into your unborn child. This energy is helping to create the cells of the stomach. The spiritual stomach is in sympathy with the love and kindness you show your unborn child. Take a deep breath in, and feel contentment pass over your body. Relax and listen to the sound of contentment, which is the sound of the note of C and the sound of the stomach.

Large Intestine

While toning a note of D, visualize the emotion of being worthy. Feel a true happiness with yourself, your spirit, and the spirit of your unborn child. Let go of all past difficulties, and look into a place of true joy. The large intestine cleanses the body. Feel it cleansing any stress, fear, and difficulty. Feel at peace. Relax and listen to the sound of self-worth, the sound of the large intestine.

Gallbladder

While toning a note of E, visualize an unborn child free of all bitterness, one with God, and entering into a world of joy and happiness. The gallbladder helps to digest food. Feel the gallbladder in harmony with the body. Relax and listen to the sound of the gallbladder.

Return now to the entire scale. Sound the notes of the scale three times, feeling the emotional harmony in your unborn child. Feel the child's peace with the world, and bring this into your world. Relax and breathe deeply, feeling the sounds with your body. How beautiful and simple are the sounds of creation. Give thanks for this peace and harmony within. Give thanks for the gift of the spirit and the process of the creation of life.

Lesson 15
Lullabies and Music for the Soul

Lullabies are soft murmurs of love and peace that can be communicated to your unborn child. This communication is offered by your special unique voice. Your distinguishable voice, your thoughts, and your feelings are all influencing your unborn child. As a parent, your personal tones and frequencies are the signature voices that your child will recognize before birth. As your child grows, the tones in your voice will trigger a range of emotions, from safety to disapproval.

When you sing or hum, soft waves of sound pass through your tissue, penetrating deep into your womb. The gentle sounds of lullabies and joyous, happy tunes create a spiritual aliveness of sound waves in the womb. Between the third and fourth month of development, your unborn child hears sounds from the outside world. He/she hears your voice singing, reading, and talking. Researchers have found that children recognize songs and music that had been played to them in the womb.

Alfred Tomatis, MD, is a French physician who has devoted his life to the healing and creative effects of music and sound. He began his work in the 1950s. He found that the ear begins to develop in the tenth week of pregnancy. He has proven that the unborn child hears low-frequency sounds, the mother's rhythmic breathing, and, of course, the parents' voice. Tomatis found that at birth the newborn can't relax until he/she hears the voice of the mother. At the time, the child moves toward the mother's voice.

Dr. Thomas Verny wrote a book called *The Secret Life of the Unborn Child*. He describes scientific experiments showing that the unborn child prefers Vivaldi and Mozart during pregnancy. The baby's heart rates steadied, and kicking decreased when these classics are played.

It is not only important to play beautiful soothing music, but also it is wonderful to read the classics to your baby. The entire family should be involved in reading out loud the Bible stories or creating a loving phrase to repeat every morning. A simple prayer or morning psalm enhances listening abilities and neural development.

After your child is born, repeating the same stories, songs, and prayers has been shown to calm the child and let them feel safe and content. The following choices demonstrate a better understanding of sound and voice that help you experience another level of communication with your unborn child.

Exercise 1

Visualize the warm and safe womb. Close your eyes, and sit quietly. Cover your ears so the sounds are muffled, as if passing through the "primordial soup" of the womb. You can sit outside in a park. Listen carefully to all the variety of tones. How does your own voice sound? Differentiating the different tones is an exercise in auditory tracking. This development continues through pregnancy and into childhood. A child is not born and then begins to slowly hear. A child is beginning to hear as the cells of the ear develop. By the fourth month, your unborn child is developing listening skills and is listening to you.

Exercise 2

Toning is a sound rather than music or song. A simple way to tone is to create a sliding scale from low notes to high notes. This sound can be a hum or a vowel or an "Aaahhh." Your voice and its wonderful range of sound that speaks out interact with the different densities of the tissues in your body. As you tone, place your hands on different areas of your body. Feel how the different low and high notes can be felt like a vibration in your organs. Generally the lower the sound, the lower you will feel it in your body. Low notes can be felt in your abdomen, and high notes can be felt in your upper chest. Practice feeling sound as it passes through your tissue and hearing sound as you create different tones with your voice.

Exercise 3

The following list may help you choose a wonderful story to read to your unborn child, or a piece of music that you will both enjoy. The sounds your child hears, even if a bit muffled, should be sweet music to their ears, creating comfort and contentment. Always remember your intention is important, and your thoughts project. Choose a favorite children's book, a bible story, a beautiful lullaby, the Lord's Prayer, a shalom chant, an alleluia chant, an om or Aum chant, a Gregorian chant, gospel music, church hymns or classical music, Vivaldi, Mozart, *The Nutcracker* suite, Bach, Handel, Corelli, Haydn, baroque music, Schubert, Schumann, Tchaikovsky, Chopin, and Liszt.

Exercise 4

Getting ready for birthing with sound is a wonderful way to relax with your child and communicate a welcoming excitement with a safe and secure supported environment of soft sound waves.

In the Oxford Journals (Volume 18, Issue 2, 1981), *Journal of Music Therapy*, Michael E. Clark, Ronald R. McCorkle, and Sterling B. William stated, "Music stimulation increases endorphin release and this decreases the need for medication. It also provides a distraction from pain and relieves anxiety." Researcher Jayne M. Standley, PhD, discovered that music played in the neonatal intensive care unit improves oxygen saturation levels, increases weight gain, shortens the hospital stay (JAMA 2000).

Creating a birthing CD is a personal and special way to bond with your child before and during birth. Choose a CD of beautiful music. A nice choice would be a baroque or classical piece. Write a short calming greeting, like in the example below. When you have created your tape, listen to it over and over again while you meditate. Close your eyes, lying down in a comfortable position, and listen to the music with your voice recorded gently talking to your child. Send your child the breath of life and unconditional love. You can create a peaceful CD with loving phrases such as the following:

- I am healthy and joyful.

- I am in a safe environment; my baby is peaceful and safe.

- I am filled with love and joy, and everyone welcomes you into this world.

- God is with us always. Let blessings and grace be with you on your journey through the birth canal.

- God, Christ, and the Holy Spirit guide your life.

- Your Father and I are with you, sending you unconditional love.

- We pray for your birth to be easy peaceful, stress–free, and quick.

- The world has been waiting for you and welcomes you in love.

- God, Christ, and the Holy Spirit are directing your birth process, and I am grateful for the love of God during my pregnancy.

The Importance of Breath

Lesson 16
Breath of Life

The sacredness of breath has always been a vital part of spiritual philosophy for centuries. It is the link that joins spirit to our physical bodies. As we take in each breath, we absorb wavelengths of life-giving energy. This energy feeds our cells with oxygen and allows us to breathe out carbon dioxide (waste products).

With each breath, we enliven our physical, emotional, mental, and spiritual bodies. In Indian prana techniques and other meditative Eastern cultures, each breath links us with the divine and the universe. In these cultures, breath is a vital part of sacred prayer.

As we breathe in, our intention and awareness of this breath focuses our energies and alters our experiences.

Dr. Marcel Vogel—an IBM senior scientist—in the early 1980s was researching breath with intention. He discovered we could focus our energies with intention and this breath of life. He did an experiment with water. He placed water into a spectrophotometer to measure absorption of wavelengths passing through the water. When he blessed the water by breathing in the love of God, love of Christ, and love of the Holy Spirit and sending that breath with intention into the water, he found two new spectral wavelengths in the now-blessed water sample. Could this be associated with the religious teaching that teaches us to pray before meals?

Blessing our food and drink adds greater absorption of energies than just thoughtlessly eating. Our gifts from God unfold as we become more conscious of our interaction with sacred energies.

In Eastern and Western medicine, the breath of life, which is twelve to sixteen times a minute, is described as the flow of cerebrospinal fluid up and down our spinal column. This breath expresses itself in the movement of (CSF) fluid, which bathes our brain every moment of life. This spinal column is also described as the Kundalini energy as it rises up the spine, through the chakra system, supporting all our tissue and energy fields of life.

Lesson 16 - Chart 1

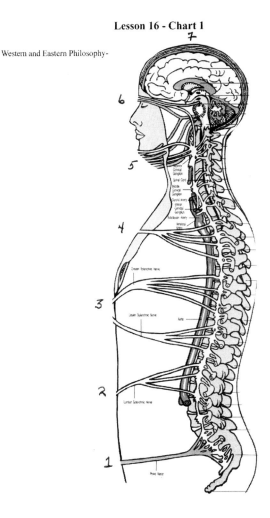

Western and Eastern Philosophy-

The following diagram describes this energy process. The areas on the chart are both locations of nerve plexus (Western scientific) as they exit the spinal column. These are physical and the ancient philosophy of chakras, which are energy maps. These are how ancient (Eastern nonscientific) humanity described our spiritual body.

Western Philosophy, Spinal Location, and Nerve Plexus: Physical Tissue

1. S4—root or base of the spinal coccygeal plexus
2. L1—lumbar-splenic plexus
3. T8—solar plexus–celiac plexus
4. C8–T1—heart or cardiac plexus
5. C3—pharyngeal plexus
6. C1—brow-carotid plexus
7. Top of head-pituitary-thalamus-brain

Eastern Philosophy and Description and Chakras: Energy

1. Etheric or physical energy
2. Astral or emotional energy
3. Lower mental bodies—math and logic
4. Higher mental bodies—creativity and relationships
5. Soul level
6. C1—spiritual knowledge and intuition
7. Spiritual—connection to God consciousness

The breath creates a wave of light energy that flows like an ocean wave up the spine, crashing on the shores of the brain, bathing our cells in the light and love of God. Your unborn child is one with the very rhythm of your breath. The ebb and flow of fluids around your child swirl about with the abdominal breathing and movement. Your child feels this movement like a gentle cradle rocking twelve to sixteen times a minute with your breath. As you breathe deeply, feel the abdomen move gently, and send that breath of light and love into the womb to bathe your child in the energy of life.

Breathing Exercise

Breathe gently into your womb. If your partner is with you, have him breathe with you and with intention, and then slowly exhale. Fill your womb with the breath of life and the pink color of unconditional love. As you close your eyes, breathe and visualize the base of your spine, and breathe deeply into the first chakra. *Chakra* means "wheel of energy" in Sanskrit. It is the chakra of physical energy. Breathe in life and health, and breathe out any tensions and physical stress.

Breathe in again, and visualize an internal space about two inches below the belly button. Breathe in emotional calm and gentle unconditional love and nurturing. This is the chakra of emotional energy, also called the lumbar-splenic plexus. Breathe in again, and visualize an internal space about two inches below the opening of the ribs. This is the chakra of mental energy, the energy of math, science, and logic. Breathe in clarity of thought. Breathe in again, and visualize your heart. This is the chakra of mental energy, the energy of creativity, language, art, and loving relationships.

Breathe in unconditional love. Breathe in again, and visualize your throat. This is the chakra of your soul. It is the energy of speaking out and following God's purpose for your soul. As you breathe in, know that you are here in divine order and that it is divine order that you and your mate have received this gift of life. Breathe in again, and visualize your brow. This is the chakra of your intuition. It is the mother's knowing and sensing area. Breathe in, and open your senses to intuit your child. Feel the love your child brings to you and your family. Breathe in again, and visualize the top of your head. This chakra is your spiritual connection to God. As you breathe in, feel the link of the life-giving breath as it connects the Holy Spirit in you to the consciousness of God. Feel this link when you pray and when you breathe. Give thanks for this sacred breath. Complete this breathing exercise with a deep cleansing breath, filling your body and your womb with the love of God. Release this breath, and send out any physical, emotional, mental, or spiritual stress, releasing any anxiety from your body and your energy fields. Breathe in, and feel the cleanliness.

The Subtle Energy of the Universe

Lesson 17
Kabbalah: Angels and Their Sacred Path

Angels have existed throughout history. They are otherworldly messengers, protectors, and sacred guides to our personal path. Paintings and writings have tried to express the spiritual nature of these incredible beings. This lesson describes their interaction with the unborn child as spirit becomes form.

In Genesis, when Adam left the garden of Eden, it is the Jewish belief that he was given information, or a type of map, that was the key to return to paradise. This Kabbalah, which translates as "received," was a pathway from the physical realm into the spiritual realm. This map was kept as oral tradition, from rabbi to rabbi, until in the 1400s, a rabbi Moses De Leon wrote it down, making it available to everyone. It was written in Hebrew, which is the alphabet of Flames, the writing of Light, which, in the Hebrew religion, is the alphabet of God.

This pathway from spirit into form is the same pathway we each take when our spirit comes from the unmanifest into the manifest, or when spirit becomes physical form. This ancient map attempts to describe our spiritual journey.

On this journey from the Great Void, the limitless light of God, we, through God, are created in the womb and brought into the Earth kingdom. Our spirit receives waves of conscious energy in the form of wisdom, understanding, loving kindness, strength, beauty, victory, splendor, formation, and, finally, physical manifestation. Along this journey, there are assigned spiritual guides, archangels, elohim, choirs of angels, and sounds (Hebrew letters). Consciousness like a wave; it pushes downward to express itself as physical matter. This energy of spirit or cosmic dust permeates and creates the expression of life through physical form.

Traveling down this wave of light is the path our spirit takes, and your unborn child is now taking to its earthly kingdom.

The gift of Kabbalah, received by humanity, is a sacred path that symbolically describes how we are formed. It also describes how our spiritual body expresses itself in physical form. This ancient (approximately six thousand years old) philosophy is still studied worldwide by the Hebrew scholars.

Kabbalah Meditation

In your womb, the incoming spirit of your unborn child travels from afar, transforming waves of light into waves of matter. Spiritual, mental, emotional, and physical form blends into multiple layers of consciousness. These layers of consciousness are guided by angelic hosts moving with spirit. There are three layers of unmanifest: Ain, Ain Soph, and Ain Soph Aur.

Through one point in time and space, the energy reaches keter, the manifestation of energy—the crown, the top of the head—and translates as "holy living ones," the direct connection between yourself and God. The archangel Metatron governs this experience and directs the energy to chokmah. Chokmah represents the force and wisdom of the soul, which is in the throat area of your body. It also translates as "wheels." Choukmah means that everything in the world reflects God's wisdom. The archangel Ratziel guides the spirit through wisdom to Binah, which is "understanding," and the archangel Tzaphkiel. These two levels, wisdom and understanding, unite at an area over the heart, which is called daat, which is knowledge. This is the journey of spirit.

Spirit pours forth into the realms of the mental bodies. The mental body heart reflects the heart area of the body and chesed, which is "loving kindness," and gevurah, which is strength. The archangels of the upper mental bodies are Tzadkiel and Kahmael. The mental body solar plexus reflects the mental concept of beauty, and its door is opened by the archangel Raphael. It is called Tiferet and is our center point, our balance point. This is the journey of the mental body aspect of spirit. The emotional body is the next unfolding for the spirit of God. It is called netzach—which is "victory," and of the archangel Uriel—and hod, which is "splendor" and of the archangel Michael. These two levels pour their light into the area of the second chakra—the emotional chakra, the neurological supply to the reproductive system in Western medicine.

At this transforming point in yesod, the actual location of the second chakra, the foundation begins to bring about physical manifestation. Yesod is the energy to the womb and is directed by the archangel Gabriel. This is the journey of the emotional body aspects of spirit. The physical formation of tissues, bones, organs, and nerves occurs at malkut. The archangel is Sandalphon. This force of light and all that has been described unites in the divine order and wisdom of God creating your special child. This unique DNA has been brought forth to express spirit in physical form.

Lesson 17 - Chart 1

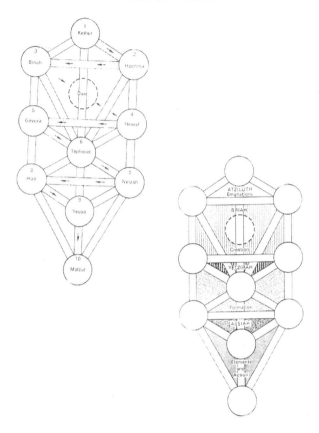

In this ancient philosophy, we can observe a map that has been studied for centuries by scholars from every religion. Our knowledge of angels has come from the ancient Hebrew scrolls. As you look at this chart, think of all the angels that guide your loving unborn child at this time. Angels guide each of us daily. Let us be thankful that God, Christ, and the Holy Spirit have created a universe of loving beings that help guide us on our life's journey.

Lesson 18
Myth and Magic of the Stars

At the moment of conception, our spirit creates a field of life energy that enlivens the womb to bring forth the creation of life. At the moment of birth, our first breath links our spirit to the physical world. Our position in the universe is defined, and our earthly journey begins. A part of our spirit has passed through the stars and planets to become alive with the breath of God. Our breath holds our spirit in the physical until that moment of our last breath, when we release our soul and journey back to our source.

The understanding of our place and our interaction with the stars and planets has been and still is a major scientific quest. As the soul enters into astrological time, it is floating in a sea of wavelengths that influence its journey. Ancient symbols of astrology are a part of our religions. We have built ziggurats, towers, or gigantic pyramids to reach between heaven and earth.

In Exodus, Moses was knowledgeable of the sacredness of all of God's creation and had the Hebrew tribes camp in the wilderness in a planetary map. This awareness of the universe was a display symbolically for the placement for the Ark of the Covenant, which was a creation of sacred space to bring God consciousness to earth. Each of the twelve tribes represented a zodiac symbol. They camped in the pattern of the stars, each tribe joined to represent all of the energies of the universe, and in the center was the Ark, the presence of God.

Lesson 18 - Chart 1

Biblical Description of the Hebrew Camp -

Asher-Aquarius

Dan- Capricorn   Naphtali- Pisces

Benjamin-Sagittarius   Judah- Aries

Menasseh-Scorpio   The Ark   IssacharTaurus

Ephraim-Libra   Zebulum-Gemini

Gad-Virgo   Reuben-Cancer

Simeon-Leo

Together this represented the God consciousness of the universe. Aaron, the high priest and Moses's brother, wore a breastplate of twelve stones, each to represent a tribe. When Aaron went into the holiest of holies to go before God, he wore this breastplate to represent all the energies of the universe. The breastplate had so much sacred energy that the Romans and the Christians also had a breastplate. Today these ancient influences are still available as birthstones. Each stone has its own absorption spectra described in science as a wavelength in the electromagnetic spectrum. Each symbolically represents the energies of the zodiac, combining to create a blend of frequencies to represent the universe and our physical bodies.

Lesson 18 - Chart 2

Exodus-Stones of The Breastplate	Apostles-Breastplate	Roman-Breastplate
Sardus, Cornelian Cancer	Andrew-Sapphire January	Garnet
Topaz Leo	Bartholomew-Cornelian February	Amethyst
Carbuncle,Ruby Virgo	James-Chalcedony March	Bloodstone
Emerald Aries	James the Less-Topaz April	Sapphire
Sapphire Taurus	John-Emerald May	Agate
Diamond Gemini	Matthew-Amethyst June	Emerald
Ligurion, Jacinth Capricorn	Matthias-Chrysolite July	Onyx
Agate Aquarius	Peter-Jasper August	Cornelian
Amethyst Pisces	Philip-Sardonyx September	Chrysolite
Chrysolite Libra	Simeon-Pink Hyacinth October	Aquamarine
Onyx Scorpio	Thaddeus-Chrysoprase November	Topaz
Jasper Sagittarius	Thomas-Beryl December	Ruby

The Breastplate Stones

Upon looking at the above charts, the interpretation and the list of stones is varied. The correspondence to specific astrological symbols also changes with time. As you review your Bible, you can read Exodus and Revelations 21 and 22. In Revelations, these stones build a structure. In the center of the structure is a river with a tree of life, which produced its own light. (Each stone produces a wavelength of light associated with it, and the wavelengths of these stones were identified by Dr. Marcel Vogel, IBM). This tree had twelve manners of fruit and yielded fruit every month. The leaves of this tree were the healers of all nations.

For centuries, astrology was pushed aside and considered unscientific. In 1955, an emission from Jupiter (long and short waves) was discovered by Burke and Franklin. Today we can identify radio waves emitted by all the planets. From Mercury to Saturn, the radiation is known as superthermals. Ultraviolet radiation is associated with Uranus, Neptune, and Pluto.

As our spiritual energy—our life force that is an energy field—enters this solar system, do we "absorb" these wavelengths? As we enter our physical bodies at birth, could these frequencies have a lasting imprint? Do we enter and absorb specific superthermals? There is not a question that they penetrate us, but there is a question of how these wavelengths interact with our physical tissue.

Recent research also shows chick embryos receive waves from the sun, which determine hatching times precisely. It was also discovered that blood coagulation is related to the phases of the moon, which means these invisible energies are shifting our tissues!

One of the greatest scientific minds of this century was Albert Einstein. He said the following:

> Astrology is a science in itself and contains an illuminating body of knowledge. It taught me many things, and I am greatly indebted to it. Geophysical evidence reveals the power of the stars and the planets in relation to the terrestrial. In turn, astrology reinforces this power to some extent. This is why astrology is like a life-giving elixir for mankind.

Meditation-Visualization

Relax with your unborn child, sitting in a comfortable location, possibly outside in the sun or in your sacred space. Close your eyes, and feel the waves of light warm your skin. Feel the waves of light touch your face, hands, and womb. These energies are all around us, and they interact with our tissue. Think of energies beyond our sun. The energies of the heavens are pouring forth all their creation and penetrating your womb, supporting the spirit and life of the child within you.

Visualize your unborn child, bathed in sunlight and heaven's creative energies. The reflections of our Creator are in everything we see. The chart of breastplate stones is symbolic of all the wavelengths of the universe. Visualize all these beautiful colored stones and their biblical history. This visualization may fill your womb with all the energies of these sacred light-producing stones, which are listed in the Bible. As you visualize the stones and their colors of light, know that these ancient creations are a part of our sacred literature.

Begin with the purple color of amethyst, and breathe into your womb the energy of purple. This multifaceted stone absorbs all colors, except purple. It reflects outward a deep purple ray of light. Next, breathe in the green color of emeralds. Send this energy into your womb, and make your child float in the life energy of green. Sapphire is the color of blue waters. Breathe gently into the womb the vibrant blues of the ocean and the color of sapphire. Diamonds are clear and bright, like the rays of the sun. They reflect all colors. Visualize white light when you breathe in the energy of diamonds. This multifaceted gemstone is like solidified white light. Sardius and cornelian are of a dark brick-red color. Breathe in the deep red of cornelian and sardius. Topaz is an orange-yellow multifaceted gemstone. The colors orange and yellow are related to thinking and intelligence. Breathe in a bright orange-yellow energy into your uterus. Ruby is a bright-red gemstone that increases your energy as you breathe its energies into your body. The color red is a very stimulating and energizing color. Breathe in the color of rubies.

Chrysolite and beryl are a dark-green serpentine stone. Breathe in the dark greens of the forest into your body, bathing the baby in the energies of peaceful evergreens. Onyx is a dense black color. It absorbs all color and reflects outward a color of dark deep space. Visualize onyx energy, and breathe in the farthest reaches of the heavens. Jasper is a dark green with red blotches in the matrix. Breathe in the colors of life-giving blood red and the dark green of pine trees. Feel the energies of jasper. This green spotted stone combines wavelengths to energize your child. Jacinth today is called zircon. Zircon is similar visually to diamonds. Breathe in the clear white light of zircon. Surround your body with all the colors of the rainbow. Agate is a rock in the family of quartz. The agate described in the Bible is moss agate. Moss agate is a clear stone with tiny green moss embedded in the matrix of the stone. As you look into the stone, you see what appears to be a small branch of moss with a solidified clear drop of rainwater on top. Breathe in the sweet green of forest moss with the clear white of rainwater quartz.

As you breathe in the energies of these biblical stones, feel them as waves of color that enlivens and penetrates your tissue. Visualize these colors; bathe your child in the energies that reflect all of humanity. Give thanks for the wonderful colors, which are the rays of light that create our world.

The study of these symbols of the universe are not only energies of specific rocks but have also been described as symbols of the biblical tribes of Israel. The theory is that we are created in the image of God, and this image is reflected in the heavens and in our bodies.

This chart represents the ancient universal influences at different times of the year.

Lesson 18 - Chart 3

Stones of Revelations-

Jasper	Sapphire	Chalcedony	Emerald	Sardonyx
Sardius	Chrysolyte	Beryl	Topaz	Chrysoprasus
Jacinth	Amethyst			

Each area of the heavens corresponds to an area of our physical bodies. The following visualization will bring the energies of the heavens into your growing and developing child. In visualization, in this meditation, the energy of the geometries of each constellation will send forth an energy to enliven your unborn child as he/she develops inside you.

Symbol	Time of Year	Planet	Body Part
Aries	3-21_4-20	Mars	Head
Taurus	4-21_5-20	Venus	Mouth and Throat
Gemini	5-21_6-21	Mercury	Lungs-Breath
Cancer	6-22_7-22	Moon	Breast and Stomach nurturing
Leo	7-23_8-22	Sun	Heart-relationships
Virgo	8-23_9-22	Mercury	Intestines-filtration
Libra	9-23_10-22	Venus	Kidneys-equilibrium
Scorpio	10-23_11-22	Pluto & Mars	Genitals and Anus-reproduction and elimination
Sagittarius	11-22_12-20	Jupiter	Hips and Thighs
Capricorn	12-21_1-19	Saturn	Bones, Skeletal, Joints
Aquirius	1-20_2-19	Uranus & Saturn	Circulatory System-Blood
Pisces	2-20_3-20	Neptune & Jupiter	Lymphatic System

Visualize the constellations in and feel the energy of the heavens, flowing through this shape and into your womb. This will help to connect you and your unborn child to the light and love of the heavens that God has created.

- Aries: Bring in the light and love of the heavenly bodies into the womb to help nourish the head and body of yourself and your unborn child.

- Taurus: Breathe in the light and love of the heavenly bodies into the womb to help nourish the mouth and throat of your body and the unborn child that you carry.

- Gemini: See the light and love of the heavenly bodies above, and connect with the universe, breathing in these sacred energies into your lungs and then deep into your womb and your child's young developing lungs.

- Cancer: Breathe into your nurturing breasts and stomach the energies of the constellation that symbolically represents them. Breathe in the love of the heavens and all of God's creations, understanding we are all one.

- Leo: Breathe into your heart love and the joy of this new relationship and this new soul entering into your family. This constellation symbolizes relationships and how important they are in your life. Breathe in the love of all your family and friends who honor and respect the soul of your unborn child, and send that love deep into your womb as you visualize this constellation.

- Virgo: Breathe into your intestines the energy of the geometries of the heavens that have represented these organs for centuries. The intestines filter and purify and bring nurturing nutrients back into the body. Feel the energy of the heavens pouring forth the rays of energy that are in harmony with your child's newly forming intestines.

- Libra: The shape of the constellation of Libra represents equilibrium and balance. This energy balances your body and is energetically connected to the organs known as the kidneys. Breathe in the light and love of God into your kidneys, and feel a peaceful balance come over your body. Breathe again deep into the womb, and ask your child to relax and feel the peace of the heavens.

- Scorpio: Scorpio energy relates to the organs of reproduction and elimination. The energy of this geometric symbolizes the energy of creation. The maleness and femaleness of your child and the creative energies of your womb are brought forth in this visualization. Breathe in the light and love of God that transforms spirit into form in your womb, and give thanks for the experience of pregnancy.

- Sagittarius: The hips and thighs are related to the stars of Sagittarius. Breathe in the light and love of movement as you meditate on this geometric symbol.

- Capricorn: Breathe in the love of God, and send this love deep into your bones and joints. This constellation brings an energy of harmony to the early growth of the small soft skeletal system of your unborn child. Breathe in this harmony into your own bones and joints, feeling the soft flexibility and strength of this tissue. Give thanks to the Creator of all things for the blessings of your pregnancy experience.

- Aquarius: Breathe in the light and love of God. Picture in your mind the geometry of the stars of the Aquarius constellation. This energy represents the energy of the blood of life. Feel the heavens above streaming this energy from deep space through the Aquarius constellation and into your circulatory system. Visualize this healthy and harmonious blood flow through you and into your unborn child. Give thanks for the blessings of this life-giving fluid.

- Pisces: Take in a deep relaxing breath. With this breath, visualize the light of the universe surrounding you and your unborn child. Look at the Pisces star constellation, and breathe into your body a cleansing energy. Pisces represents the lymphatic system, which is your cleansing system. The red blood cells bring nutrients to the tissue and the lymph, cleansing the tissue, removing waste. Give thanks for the healing and cleansing action of the lymph and the energy this system might receive from the heavens above.

Lesson 18 - Chart 5

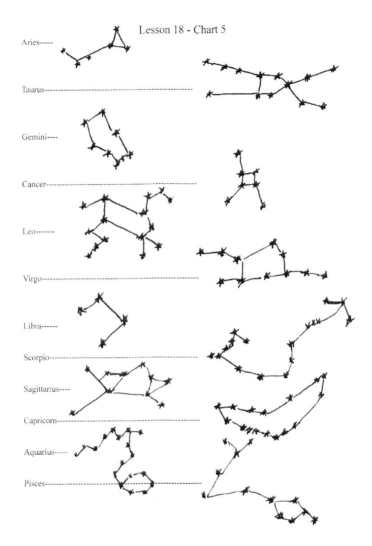

Aries-----

Taurus--

Gemini----

Cancer--

Leo--------

Virgo--

Libra------

Scorpio--

Sagittarius----

Capricorn--

Aquarius-----

Pisces--

Sacred Words

Lesson 19
Holy Names of God

In our earliest beginnings, our prehistory, we thought that our sun was God. It was named Apollo, the god of light. Venus, the morning star—which is actually a planet—symbolized love and beauty. Mercury was the divine scribe. These planets represented gods because they are in motion. They have a defined, observed path through the heavens. The stars almost appear to be a motionless backdrop to these sacred traveling beings. The patterns of stars were a map to plot the movement of the gods across the sky. The sun brought life to the day, and the moon brought life to the night.

This memory of our names of God has become part of our collective unconscious. Our physical, emotional, mental, and spiritual bodies are carrying all the DNA of our past ancestors as archetypes. Our names of the week were in ancient days, our names of God:

1. Monday: dies Lunae, day of moon, goddess of nature, intuition, mother of all things

2. Tuesday: dies Martis, day of Mars, god of war and peace

3. Wednesday: dies Mercurii, day of Mercury, messenger of the gods, symbol of power and speed

4. Thursday: dies Jovis, day of Jupiter, god of light, governs the heavens and earth

5. Friday: dies Veneris, day of Venus, goddess of love and beauty

6. Saturday: dies Saturni, day of Saturn, god of time, quest for greater awareness

7. Sunday: dies Dominica, day of Sun, god of music, the source of heat, light, and life

Our perceptions have shifted, and when we grow, we then shifted our perception of God.

Exercise 1

Each morning, when you wake up, take a few moments for a morning prayer with your unborn child. Start by quietly greeting the new day. Breathe in the breath of life, and say, "This is the day that the Lord has made. Let us rejoice and celebrate today." If it is Friday, then add, "This is Friday, the ancient day of Venus. The universe you come into is great, beautiful, and filled with love, and the planets greet you each day."

The ancient and indigenous tribes relied on shamans to speak with the spirits or the gods of creation. Not everyone was allowed to pray, meditate, or attempt to communicate with God. In the Inuit (Eskimo) philosophy, the sea was the home of powerful spirits. The Inuit creator of all the sea creatures was called

Sedna. The Inuit believed the great sea mother was always there, and the shaman's (angakok) soul would travel to this great sea mother and ask for a message. Another shift in our religious perception was that anyone can pray. In a sense, we are all shamans, capable of speaking a prayer and asking God for direction.

In ancient times, we discovered sacred sites, wells, and springs of life-giving water that had magical healing properties. This energy was so special we created stone structures at holy sites and worshipped the life-giving gifts of the earth at these sites. We worshipped the female goddess Mother Earth, the creator of all things. When the Christian religion began all over England and Europe, churches were built on these "earth energy" sacred sites. Our vision transferred from the intimate knowledge and feeling of the sacred earth as a representation of God consciousness to our personal Christian religious belief of what is God consciousness. This shifted our perception again, expanding our perception of God.

The ancient Greek school of philosophy attempted to describe the science of god. Anaxagoras described God to be the divine infinite mind, not enclosed in any body.

Our perceptions changed again, from feeling God in the earth and in all living creatures to trying to describe our observations of the creation in scientific terms.

Pythagoras of Samos (Pythagoras lived between 580 BC and 500 BC) looked at God's creation, the universe, and studied the math of existence. Each planet had a math proportion, a musical note, a sound as it flew through the ethers of the heavens. Pythagoras used the same proportions as God and created the string instrument called a lyre. He discovered these musical notes could create emotions and described musical medicine. All of creation is a divine mathematical map.

Exercise 2

Begin with a gentle silence that relaxes all your cells. Sound the musical scale with a hum, rising slowly from a very low deep note to the highest note you can reach. You are sounding the notes of creation, our musical scale. If you are uncomfortable humming or singing, use a musical instrument, if it is available. Look into your womb, and silently, quietly listen to hear the music of creation in your womb. If you cannot hear it, then relax further and try to feel it in your soul. Look up toward the stars and planets tonight. Listen and feel the vibrations and music of the spheres. This same experience inspired Pythagoras to create music.

Abraham, the father of the Jewish and Islamic religions, was one of the first to have a concept of one god over all creation. One Creator! In Genesis, the name of God was a Hebrew word called Elohim, which is defined as a plural god, a messenger of God. Abraham evolved mankind to shift our perceptions again into a definition of one God, the Creator. Organized religion has as many names for God as there are languages. Gandhi once said, "If we have listening ears, God speaks to us in our own language, whatever that language is." Today, scientists are mapping a language of creation with genetics, but this will be a detailed physical map;

it does not describe the essence of God consciousness. Scientists will try to state that DNA is the essence of our creation, but we are greater than the physical representation of our tissue.

This next exercise opens your heart to understanding the many concepts of God. As one people of earth, we each contain a breath of holy life, a timeless, spaceless essence of the Holy Spirit of God. It is a manifestation of love to understand another's deepest belief. We as holy spirits have experienced many religions to describe the spiritual essence of our Creator. Feel the closeness and love you have for your unborn child. This can only describe a fraction of the love your Creator has for you. To sound the name of God with intention brings you into a harmony with the energies of creation. During your pregnancy, it is important to fill your body and your unborn child with not only a healthy diet, exercise, and positive thoughts but also with your personal perception of the energy of God consciousness. People have experienced God through prayer, meditation, visions, and dreams. Speaking and feeling the energy of the holy names of God brings into you a greater understanding of the feeling of God in your world. The following list evokes an energy of creation that these words cannot speak.

Exercise 3

Bring the energy of the Creator into your womb. As you silently feel the subtle energy of life, you can feel how millions of people, for centuries, have chanted the sacred words to express God. These chants and prayers have been spoken in many languages. They have been spoken with intention in all areas of our world. These words have, to each individual, meant the same thing: one God, the Creator of all things. Sit in a relaxed position and speak these words slowly and clearly. As you speak these sacred words, close your eyes and feel the subtle energy of the love of each religion. The intention of honoring all beliefs without judgment is the first step to sending this wonderful energy of God into the sacred space of your womb. This list is not complete. If your religious perception of God is not listed, add this sacred name to top of this list. Repeat this list at least three times to feel this subtle energy of the names of God. Give thanks for the variety of love of spirit alive today.

1. God, Jesus Christ, Holy Spirit- Christianity,

2. Allah- Islam

3. Ain Soph- Kabbalah, Mystical Judaism

4. Brahma- Hinduism

5. Ahurra Mazda-Zoroastria nism, Ancient Persia

6. Yud-Hei-Vov-Hei- Judaism

7. Jehovah-Judaism and Christianity

8. Adonia Judaism

This list is incomplete but only offered to share the love of the Creator and the honor and respect of others' religious views. Feel the love all the peoples of earth have for God. Feel the joy of unconditional love, which is a blessing from Christ.

Lesson 20
First Sounds and Sacred Tones

Sacred languages were created for divine communication. The idea of expressing sounds to communicate with spirit is ancient. This experience is a common thread through all religions and philosophies. This lesson describes the sounds that begin with creation. Creation is occurring at this moment within your womb. Divine energy patterns appear to silently unfold, creating a child who will soon express him/herself as a part of the breath of God. This lesson will connect you and your unborn child with the sounds and symbols of creation.

Hebrew

The word *Hebrew* is defined as "a sign or heavenly revelation." The mystical study of Kabbalah believes that the twenty-two letters of the Hebrew alphabet created the whole of creation past, present, and future. An understanding of matter that is beyond our perceptions could be achieved by mastering the Hebrew sounds. Just as we have found the DNA—the code of life—the Kabbalists felt the letters were the vibrational codes of the formation of the universe. Sounds are a key pathway to shift our energy fields. Just as music creates happiness, joy, or the blues, these simple vibrations give us an understanding of the first sounds of creation. Even if you speak absolutely no Hebrew, you can sound the letters and ask the Creator of all things to form them into energy patterns that will uplift your family, yourself, and your unborn child. Each person, just like each sound, has a unique purpose in the divine plan. The story of the first sounds of the Hebrew alphabet is the story of creation. In the twenty-two letters, three are mother letters.

Lesson 20 - Chart 1

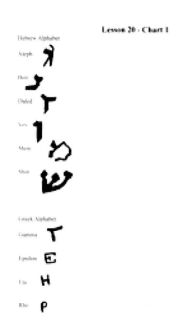

The first mother letter is *A*, aleph. Aleph makes no sound of its own when it is in a word. It projects the stillness and silence of the primal force of creation even before perception. Aleph is divine oneness. Aleph is the sound of spirit and represents the element of air. From aleph (air), another element was extracted, which is water (land and sea). This water is the sound *mem*. From water, the vibration of fire was extracted, which represents heaven and the letter *shin*. Sounds create life and movement. The first sounds of the Hebrew language should murmur thoughts of spiritual joy, oneness, peace, and creation. This short list was chosen to be utilized during meditation at this special time of pregnancy and creation. Look at the shapes of these symbols, and tone the letter, quietly feeling the energy patterns of life.

Aleph—the sound of stillness and silence, the first mother sound of all creation—is the sound of God. This divine oneness is a sound in the energy pattern before manifestation into the physical aleph combines in different vibrations, unfolding into different sounds, which are letters that create the seen and the unseen worlds. It represents the air or the breath of life.

Beit is associated with a house of the divine. At this moment, your womb of fertility is the sacred dwelling for the spirit and soul of your unborn child. In this divine house, there is peace and love. Nourish your child's environment with the gentle vibrations of beit. Beit begins the word *blessings*. As you speak this letter, think of all the blessings you receive.

Daled is considered the sound of pregnancy and creation. The process of creation or the manifestation of spiritual energy into physical form has a specific energy process that has been mapped by the Kabbalist. Everything that we see has journeyed from the upper levels of the unmanifest (limitless light) through the four realms of the universe:

1. Aziluth: emanation—energy of the divine (spiritual body)

2. Berial: creation—ideas and thoughts formless (mental body)

3. Yetirah: formation—the blueprints of physical reality without physical reality

4. Assiyah: action—the energy, matter, and physical reality in which we live.

At this time, spiritual doorways are opened by the sound of daled, bringing in the creation of your unborn child at every moment until the doorway of birth has opened, and you are blessed with the care of God's new creation.

Vov, the sixth letter of the alphabet, represents physical wholeness and the uniqueness of each person's spiritual path. As you sound this letter, honor the special spiritual path of your unborn child.

As you sound the letter mem, try to perceive the sound of the earth, the land, and the sea. Mystically, the letter mem represents human consciousness and the watery realms of spirit. This realm is our access to spiritual communication. Mem is the beginning letter of the Hebrew word for *angel* (moloch), which means "messenger." As you sound mem, ask to open the channels of spiritual communication if it is God's purpose for you at this time.

Shin represents the element of fire, which also represents the heavens. Shin is the beginning letter of the word *shalom*, which is "peace." As you complete this meditation, feel the spiritual peace of the sound of shin. As you tone this sound, feel it permeate your womb with the peace of God.

The Greek Alphabet

There are many myths concerning the origins of the Greek alphabet. Greek is considered a sacred language because it represents a subtle esoteric interrelationship between symbols, numbers, and letters. This interrelationship consciously evolves us into a greater understanding of the world, a gnosis, which is intuitive knowledge. As you create the sounds of the Greek letters, think of their meanings and feel the gnosis. or knowledge of ancient truths that are represented by these sacred tones.

Gamma is the third letter of the Greek alphabet. It represents the number 3, and from the sacredness of creation from the mother and father comes the child. This trinity is in every religion: the Egyptians worshipped Isis, Osiris, and Horus. The Vikings worshipped Odin, Thor, and Balder. The Babylonians worshipped Anu, Enlil, and Ea. The trinity is in nature: birth, life, and death; and creation, continuance, and destruction. Sound the letter gamma, and feel the energies of the trinity. Feel the energies of yourself and your husband blending together on multiple levels, creating this special spiritual being, your unborn child.

Epsilon is the subtle energy of life. This tone is the spiritual energy of matter that is within your child now. This subtle energy is like a field of energy that bathes your child's physical, emotional, and mental growth. This energy is represented as a five-pointed star, and it is the energy of form, a sacred form that is called sacred geometry. These ancient geometries were used to design the most sacred structures: the Parthenon in Athens and the temple of Zeus at Olympia. As you sound epsilon, feel the energy of spirit in the physical world. Feel the energy of design in all living things. Breathe in deeply, and feel the energy of epsilon in your own perfectly designed body.

Eta, the seventh character of the Greek alphabet, represents joy and love. It is the quality of being in total harmony with the world, which is divine harmony. Send your child joy and love by toning Eta. Visualize your child and your womb as being filled with joy and love. Feel this love bring divine harmony and a sense of completion into your family at this time. This special child brings joy, love, and harmony, which creates spiritual balance, bringing everyone closer to the divine energies of life.

Rho is the seventeenth letter of the Greek alphabet. Rho represents creativity, fruitfulness, growth, and reproduction. It is the feminine qualities that are in both male and female. It is the creative energy that brings forth form. It is the journey of becoming. The letter rho is the creation and energy of your unborn child as he/she comes into being. As you tone rho, feel the journey of pregnancy and the journey of your unborn child, and give thanks for this wonderful experience of reproduction.

Look through a favorite language and find the sacred sounds. Find the sacred sounds of nature—a waterfall, a songbird, a child's laugh. These are the sounds of creation that we can experience every day with great joy and blessings.

Spirit

Lesson 21
Gifts of the Spirit

This Holy Spirit, this essence of God that enlivens our physical tissue, also enlivens our hearts. Our interaction and relationships with others and our environment is our consciousness of the spirit of God in us. This was eloquently said by the apostle Paul, in a letter to the Corinthians. In this passage, he beautifully described the gifts of the spirit that we each receive at conception as the spirit of life begins to stir in the womb.

> Now there are diversities of gifts, but the same spirit. And there are differences of administrations, but the same Lord. And there are diversities of operations, but it is the same Lord which worketh all in all. But the manifestation of the spirit is given to every man to profit withal. For to one is given by the spirit the word of wisdom; to another the word of knowledge by the same spirit; To another faith by the same spirit; to another the gifts of healing by the same spirit; To another the working of miracles; to another prophecy; to another discerning of spirits; to another divers kinds of tongues; to another the interpretation of tongues: But all there worketh that one and the self-same spirit, dividing to every man

severally as he will. For as the body is one, and hath many members, and all the members of that one body, being many, are one body: so also is Christ. For by one spirit we are all baptized into one body, whether we be Jew or Gentiles, Whether we be bond or free; and have been made to drink from one spirit. For the body is not one member, but many.

1 Corinthians 12:4–12:14

In this passage, Paul describes gifts given to each of us that shape our lives. Whether your child becomes a healer or has great knowledge, it is considered by most religions to be a gift from God. It is the essence of the same spirit that is in all of us that enters at conception and leaves at death. This spirit expresses a consciousness that understands we are all one, even if we appear in different forms or have different ideas. The breath of life that creates you and your child creates all of life. There is no separation of spirit; there is only spirit.

Meditation

After you have read the passage listing the gifts of the spirit, relax and visualize this quiet meditation. You may go to that sacred space in your home or sit outside under a favorite tree in your yard. The energy of spirit surrounds you with life at every moment; it is your choice to look around and feel this force of life. Take a slow deep breath into your body and relax. Next, take a slow breath in, and quiet your mind. Breathe deep into your womb, sending unconditional love into the welcome spirit of your child. As you breathe gently, see with your spiritual eye a joyful ceremony honoring the incoming spirit of your child. The angelic hosts have come to greet your child. The Holy Spirit has come like a dove from the heavens with a large chest. In this chest are the gifts of the Spirit. As the dove slowly opens the chest, the air smells sweet and the soft breeze swirls around your womb like a warm shawl. The music is heavenly, and it floats on the breeze, like a mist over the water. What is this magical state of peace and joy that is the Holy Spirit?

As you relax, the dove opens the chest and offers these sacred gifts to your child. Like balls of light, the energy permeates your womb and the child receives each gift of light with an unearthly joy that you feel through your entire body. Breathe in this light of spirit, this energy of life, and give thanks for the gifts your unborn child has received. Relax and stay in the moment for as long as your consciousness can feel the peace. Then open your eyes and stretch, feeling the expanded consciousness of your unborn child. This expanded consciousness is in all your fellow man. As you look around today, see all the gifts of the spirit in everyone—in your doctor, teacher, and in your family.

The Fruits of the Spirit

The passage related to 1 Corinthians is Galatians 5:22–23. In this passage, the fruits of the Spirit are described. The fruits are produced by the Spirit as it is blossoming and interacting with other spirits of the same one God consciousness. These you have experienced each day of your life, and as you interact with the spirit of your unborn child, these fruits your child will feel also.

> But the fruit of the spirit is love, joy, peace, long-suffering, gentleness, goodness, faith, meekness, temperance: against such there is no law.

Galatians 5:22–23

Of all these fruits, because the Holy Spirit is in you, you may send these fruits that you have to your unborn child. Take a deep breath in, and ask your Spirit to send love to the spirit of your unborn child. Repeat the same procedure for each fruit, and then give thanks.

Lesson 22
The Hundredth Monkey

The love we have for ourselves and our unborn children creates an expanding subtle energy field. This growing energy touches everyone. It can start with you. Here is a true story of this expanding energy field in which we are all members. The moment your unborn child brings his or her consciousness to this planet, they become a part of the earth's life consciousness. The study of these subtle energies brings you to an awareness of these energies. This story is about these subtle energies at work in our lives.

Japanese monkeys have been observed and studied in the wild for over sixty years. The Japanese monkey *Macaca fuscata* lives on the island of Koshima. In 1952, scientists were supplying monkeys with sweet potatoes. They would leave a mound of sweet potatoes each day in the dirt. The monkeys liked the taste of the raw sweet potatoes but found the dirt to be unpleasant.

One sunny morning, an eighteen-month-old female named Imo picked up her sweet potato, walked down to a nearby stream, and proceeded to wash off her sweet potato before eating it.

She taught this trick to her mother.

She taught her playmates, and they taught their mothers too.

The scientists watched this evolution. It was incredible! Between 1952 and 1958, all the young monkeys learned to wash the dirty, sandy sweet potatoes. Only the adults who imitated their children learned to eat clean sweet potatoes. The other adults kept eating the dirty sweet potatoes.

Then in the autumn of 1958, something startling took place. An unknown number of Koshima monkeys were washing their sweet potatoes. If we suppose ninety-nine monkeys had learned to wash their sweet potatoes that special morning, when the sun rose and the hundredth monkey learned how to wash a sweet potato, the most incredible consciousness evolution occurred.

By that evening, almost every monkey suddenly began washing sweet potatoes before eating them. A certain amount of monkeys were conscious, and a breakthrough occurred. A subtle energy altered the consciousness of all monkeys. Colonies of monkeys on other islands and the mainland troop of monkeys at Takasakiyama began spontaneously washing their sweet potatoes. The scientists were shocked. When a certain critical number achieves an awareness, consciousness of living beings communicate this information from mind to mind.

The hundredth-monkey phenomenon means if a limited number of mothers make a breakthrough to begin to try to spiritually communication with their unborn children, the consciousness becomes a part of all mothers, bringing the consciousness of God into our birth experience.

We have always loved and gently sung to our unborn children. Now we have shifted our subtle energy to acknowledge their soul. The consciousness shift creates a new intimate relationship between mother and child. Enjoy the many blessings you both receive.

Spiritual Connectedness

The spiritual connectedness you have at this moment in time is a closeness to God and spirit that expresses itself through creation. While you are pregnant, your awareness and senses heighten. You feel things and smell things you could never have felt or sensed. You are keenly aware of the energies around you. Realize today that the awareness of these energies is an awareness of the subtle energy of life. Know that we are all one in the consciousness of God. Sit down in a relaxed and comfortable sacred space, and be conscious of these feelings. Close your eyes, and take a few deep breaths. Breathe in the love of God into your womb. Breathe in the love of God into your body. Breathe in the love of God into your sacred space. Relax and feel the love of God as an unconditional love that nurtures all mankind. It is the love of the Holy Spirit that flows through all our lives. See that energy as rays of light touching your womb and then feel that you are one with your child.

Next, see this light fill your entire house. Quietly breathe and watch this light blanket your neighbors and then your entire community. There are pockets of people meditating and praying all over the earth, The Christians, the Jews, the Tibetan monks, and Zen masters, each in their own way, are creating pockets of light. They are trying to divine and spiritually communicate as you are with your unborn child. When enough people are in spiritual communication, the lights of these tiny pockets will blend into one. It is then that we will feel the unconditional love of God in everything we do. The interconnectedness of our spirit should bring us to a consciousness of God that will bring joy and peace to this blessed moment of pregnancy.

Your light and communication today will open channels to more light, unconditional love, and spiritual communication in our futures. Thank God for the gift of your loving child and all children. Send your unconditional love to children everywhere, knowing that your intentions will reach and nurture them on many subtle levels. We are all gifts from God. Let us take a moment to honor our gift. Take a deep breath of the fresh air that mingles in and out of all our lungs and realize we are all one.